THERAPEUTIC NEEDS
OF THE FAMILY

Publication Number 934
AMERICAN LECTURE SERIES®

A Publication in
The BANNERSTONE DIVISION *of*
AMERICAN LECTURES IN SOCIAL AND REHABILITATION
PSYCHOLOGY

Editors of the Series
RICHARD E. HARDY, Ed.D.

Chairman, Department of Rehabilitation Counseling
Virginia Commonwealth University

and

JOHN G. CULL, Ph.D.

Director, Regional Counselor Training Program
Department of Rehabilitation Counseling
Virginia Commonwealth University
Fishersville, Virginia

The American Lecture Series in Social and Rehabilitation Psychology offers books which are concerned with man's role in his milieu. Emphasis is placed on how this role can be made more effective in a time of social conflict and a deteriorating physical environment. The books are oriented toward descriptions of what future roles should be and are not concerned exclusively with the delineation and definition of contemporary behavior. Contributors are concerned to a considerable extent with prediction through the use of a functional view of man as opposed to a descriptive, anatomical point of view.

Books in this series are written mainly for the professional practitioner; however, academicians will find them of considerable value in both undergraduate and graduate courses in the helping services.

Therapeutic Needs Of the Family

Problems, Descriptions and Therapeutic Approaches

RICHARD E. HARDY, Ed.D.
JOHN G. CULL, Ph.D.

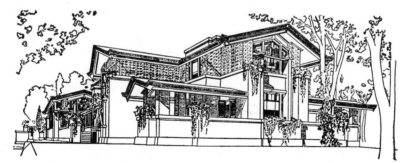

CHARLES C THOMAS · PUBLISHER
Springfield · Illinois · USA

Published and Distributed Throughout the World by

CHARLES C THOMAS • PUBLISHER

Bannerstone House

301-327 East Lawrence Avenue, Springfield, Illinois, U.S.A.

© 1974, by CHARLES C THOMAS • PUBLISHER

ISBN 0-398-03048-0

Library of Congress Catalog Card Number: 73 17045

With THOMAS BOOKS careful attention is given to all details of manufacturing and design. It is the Publisher's desire to present books that are satisfactory as to their physical qualities and artistic possibilities and appropriate for their particular use. THOMAS BOOKS will be true to those laws of quality that assure a good name and good will.

Printed in the United States of America

A-1

Library of Congress Cataloging in Publication Data

Hardy, Richard E.
    Therapeutic needs of the family.

    (American lecture series, publication no. 934.
A publication in the Bannerstone division of American
lectures in social and rehabilitation psychology)
    1. Family psychotherapy. I. Cull, John G., joint
author. II. Title. [DNLM: 1. Family therapy.
WM430 T396 1974]
RC488.5.H35   616.8'915   73-17045
ISBN 0-398-03048-0

This book is dedicated to:

WAYNE SMITH GILL, Ph.D.

warm friend and psychologist par excellence

CONTRIBUTORS

JAMES F. ALEXANDER, Ph.D., is an associate professor at the University of Utah. He is also currently coordinator of community practicum training, consultant to various agencies (Salt Lake Veterans Administration Hospital, Utah State Juvenile Court, and Salt Lake Comprehensive Community Mental Health Center). He has authored numerous journal articles and convention papers on family interaction and family therapy including *Journal of Counsulting and Clinical Psychology, Journal of Marriage and the Family.*

JOHN G. CULL, Ph.D.: Director, Regional Counselor Training Program and Professor, Department of Rehabilitation, School of Community Services, Virginia Commonwealth University, Fishersville, Va.; Adjunct Professor in Psychology and Education, School of General Studies, University of Virginia; Technical Consultant, Rehabilitation Services Administration, U. S. Department of Health, Education and Welfare; Vocational Consultant, Bureau of Hearings and Appeals, Social Security Administration; Lecturer, Medical Department Affiliate Program, Woodrow Wilson Rehabilitation Center; Consulting Editor, *American Lecture Series in Social and Rehabilitation Psychology*, Charles C Thomas, Publisher. Formerly Rehabilitation Counselor, Texas Commission for the Blind and Texas Rehabilitation Commission; Director, Division of Research and Program Development, Virginia Department of Vocational Rehabilitation. The following are some of the books Dr. Cull has co-authored and co-edited: *Vocational Rehabilitation: Profession and Process, Contemporary Fieldwork Practices in Rehabilitation, Social and Rehabilitation Services for the Blind, Fundamentals of Criminal Behavior and Correctional Systems* and *Drug Dependence and Rehabilitation Approaches.* Dr. Cull also has contributed more than 50 publications to the professional literature in psychology and rehabilitation.

E. LEE DOYLE, Ph.D.: Associate Professor, College of House-hold Arts & Sciences, Texas Womens University, Denton, Texas. Dr. Doyle also is in private practice in Dallas, Texas. Her primary areas of interests are marital and family counseling, behavioral and conditioning therapy, client therapist interaction, family therapy and psychotherapy. Formerly, Dr. Doyle was Associate Professor with the California State College, Long Beach, California; Co-therapist and Research Associate with the Reproductive Biological Research Foundation; Research Assistant, Florida State University and Assistant Professor, East Texas State University. Dr. Doyle received degrees from East Texas State University and Florida State University. She is a member of the American Psychological Association and has Divisional membership in the Division of Psychopharmacology and Division of Psychotherapy.

RICHARD E. HARDY, Ed.D.: Chairman, Department of Rehabilitation, School of Community Services, Virginia Commonwealth University, Richmond, Virginia; Technical Consultant, Rehabilitation Services Administration, U. S. Department of Health, Education and Welfare; Consulting Editor, *American Lecture Series in Social and Rehabilitation Psychology*, Charles C Thomas, Publisher; and Associate Editor, *Journal of Voluntary Action Research*. Formerly, Rehabilitation Counselor in Virginia; Chief Psychologist and Supervisor of Training, South Carolina Department of Vocational Rehabilitation and member South Carolina State Board of Examiners in Psychology, Rehabilitation Advisor, Rehabilitation Services Administration, U. S. Department of Health, Education and Welfare. The following are some of the books Dr. Hardy has co-authored and co-edited: *Social and Rehabilitation Services for the Blind, Vocational Rehabilitation: Profession and Process, The Unfit Majority, Fundamentals of Criminal Behavior and Correctional Systems* and *Drug Dependence and Rehabilitation Approaches*. Dr. Hardy has contributed more than 50 publications to the professional literature in psychology and rehabilitation.

GORDON A. HARSHMAN, Ph.D.· Associate Professor of Counseling and Guidance at the University of Arizona. He completed doctoral work in Counseling Psychology at the Ohio State University in 1963. His major interest, the improvement of interpersonal communication, takes the form of training counselors, teachers and other education specialists in using and transmitting communication skills and applications of group process in educational and other community settings. As consultant with the Counseling and Consulting Center of Tucson, he specializes in marriage and family counseling, group therapy and human relations training.

GILBERT L. INGRAM, Ph.D.: Coordinator, Mental Health Programs and Chief Psychologist, Federal Correctional Institution, Tallahassee, Florida; Adjunct Lecturer, Department of Psychology, Florida State University; Consultant, Georgia State Department of Family and Children Services, Waycross Regional Youth Development Center; Book Reviewer, Correctional Psychologist. Formerly, Chief Psychologist, Robert F. Kennedy Youth Center, Adjunct Assistant Professor, West Virginia University, Instructor, Alderson-Broaddus College, Chief Psychologist, National Training School for Boys, and Research Project Director, Federal Bureau of Prisons. Dr. Ingram also has contributed numerous articles to the professional literature in correctional psychology, crime and delinquency.

ROBERTA MALOUF: Ms. Malouf is a staff psychologist at the Granite Community Mental Health Center in Salt Lake City and a doctoral candidate in clinical psychology at the University of Utah. In addition to family therapy her research interests include psycholinguistics and child development. She has authored several convention papers and published in *Developmental Psychology* and *Child Development*.

JOSEPH N. MERTZ, A.C.S.W.: Currently Supervisor of Social Services, The Workshop, Rehabilitation Center, Menands, New York. Mr. Mertz received his B.A. and M.A. in Sociology, Siena College, Loudonville, New York, and his M.S. in Social Work, Columbia University, New York City. Formerly, with the New York State Department of Mental Hygiene in both a State Hospital setting and as Administrator of traveling Child Guidance Clinics; Chief Psychiatric Social Worker and Administrator—Community Mental Health Clinics; Supervisor of Social Services in two counties at a Family Court level. Mr. Mertz is in private practice, part-time in marriage counseling, emotional disturbances in children and adults and is consultant to clinics and social agencies on private level.

HENRY RAYMAKER, JR., Ph.D.: Chief, Psychology Service, Veterans Administration Center, Dublin, Georgia; Consultant, College Street Hospital, Macon, Georgia; Consultant, Office of Rehabilitation Services, Atlanta, Georgia; Consultant, Regional Youth Development Center, Sandersville, Georgia; Consultant, Department of Family and Children Services, Atlanta, Georgia; private practice, Dublin, Georgia. Dr. Raymaker has been a licensed clinical psychologist in the State of Georgia since 1957 and has his Ph.D. degree in clinical psychology from Vanderbilt University.

AGNES M. RITCHIE, A.C.S.W.: Instructor (social work), Department of Neurology and Psychiatry, and Chief Psychiatric Social Worker, Division of Child Psychiatry, University of Texas Medical Branch, Galveston, Texas.

JEROME ROSENBERG, Ph.D.: Assistant Professor, Department of Psychology, New College, University of Alabama, University, Alabama; Consultant, Rehabilitation Research Foundation, Draper Correctional Center, Elmore, Alabama; Consultant, Tuscaloosa Association Retarded Children's Opportunity School; Board of Directors, Tuscaloosa Association for Retarded Children, Tuscaloosa Community Crisis Center; Member, Association for the Advancement of Behavior Therapy, American Psychological Association; plus numerous other professional organizations. Formerly, Coordinator of Testing and Evaluation, University Counseling Center, Florida State University. Dr. Rosenberg has conducted numerous workshops in counseling, behavior modification and behavior therapy and is writing in the areas of his professional interest.

ALEXANDER P. RUNCIMAN, Ph.D.: Dr. Runciman is a clinical psychologist in private practice in Van Nuys, California. He received degrees from the University of Southern California. Formerly he was the first Co-Therapist to join the Masters and Johnson clinical program for sexual therapy. He was a Research Associate at the Reproduction Biology Research Foundation, St. Louis, Missouri. Prior to that Dr. Runciman was Director of the Sir Thomas Moore Clinic, Van Nuys, California. He is a certified social psychologist and is a licensed marriage, family and child counselor, with the State of California. Dr. Runciman has several articles in professional journals and currently has a book in progress.

ALBERTO C. SERRANO, M.D.: Director, Community Guidance Center, San Antonio, Texas; Associate Professor of Psychiatry in Pediatrics, University of Texas Medical School at San Antonio; Director, Child and Adolescent Psychiatry, University of Texas Medical School at San Antonio.

MARJORIE KAWIN TOOMIM, Ph.D.: Dr. Toomim received her Doctorate from the University of Southern California. She has held several positions of responsibility in the Los Angeles area. Currently Dr. Toomim is in private practice. Her areas of interests are in community psychology, child development, humanistic psychology and separation counseling.

DAVID A. VORE, Ph.D.: Dr. Vore received his Ph.D. in Clinical Psychology from Purdue University in 1969. His areas of specialization are in Clinical Child and Developmental Psychology. Dr. Vore is currently an Assistant Professor in the Department of Pediatrics and of the Department of Behavioral Sciences and Psychiatry, and Director of Pediatric Psychology at Children's Memorial Hospital of the University of Oklahoma Health Sciences Center. He is Secretary-Treasurer of the Society of Pediatric Psychology, a subsection of Section 1 of Division 12 of the American Psychological Association. Since joining the University of Oklahoma Health Sciences Center, Dr. Vore has made a major commitment to studying and working with terminally ill children and their families.

LOGAN WRIGHT, Ph.D.: Dr. Wright received his Ph.D. in Clinical Psychology from George Peabody College for Teachers in 1964. His speciality areas are Clinical Child and Developmental Psychology. Dr. Wright is currently an Associate Professor in the Department of Pediatrics and of the Department of Psychiatry and Behavioral Sciences. He has been active in the area of Pediatric Psychology and has published extensively on a number of topics.

FOREWORD

ANTHROPOLOGISTS TELL US that the most persistent institution in the history of mankind has been the family unit. The family unit has been traced as a phenomenon back to the dawn of man. The family unit has seemed to be impervious to external pressures which impinge on this unit or external pressures which impinge upon individuals within the unit. However, we are now seeing increased evidence within our culture that the family unit is no longer as impervious to pressure and change as it once was. We now are seeing many types of pressures which are weakening the solidarity of the family unit. Divorce rates are soaring not only in our country and culture but across the world. Perhaps the most persistent attacks on the family unit have centered around questions relating to the effectiveness and purpose of the family. The family no longer serves a major role in inculcating the social and moral mores of our society. Other institutions have assumed responsibility for this role. The attacks on the viability and practicality of family units commenced with the lower class families. However, the questions of the efficacy of a family unit has spread on to the middle and upper classes so that now it is a generalized concern among sociologists.

More and more psychologists and counselors are being confronted with clients whose basic problem is a deteriorating marriage and thereby the impending breakup of the family unit. In an effort to assist psychologists and counselors in understanding some of the problems and in providing some suggested approaches in working with these people, we have developed this book. We have tried to identify some of the key problems which seem to add undue stress to the family. In identifying these problems we also have to identify approaches to solutions which may be implemented through counseling approaches. It is our earnest hope that we may make a basic contribution toward increasing the viability and stability of family units experiencing crises.

We are deeply indebted to the contributors to this book for their understanding and patience, for the outstanding work they have done, and for being so kind and receptive to our many inquiries, criticisms and comments.

JOHN G. CULL
RICHARD E. HARDY

CONTENTS

THERAPEUTIC NEEDS
OF THE FAMILY

Chapter I

GROUP WORK WITH DISTRESSED FAMILIES

JOHN G. CULL AND RICHARD E. HARDY

- MARITAL ROLES IN GROUP COUNSELING
- RELATIONSHIPS NECESSARY FOR EFFECTIVE GROUP INTERACTION
- GROUND RULES FOR GROUP MARITAL SESSIONS
- TIME PERIODS AND TYPES OF SESSIONS

MARITAL ROLES IN GROUP COUNSELING

OFTEN IT IS DIFFICULT TO DISCRIMINATE between actual behavior and behavior which is related by a marriage partner. This period of counseling is difficult; the marriage counselor is interacting on a one-to-one basis or is occasionally seeing both marriage partners together. As a result of the defensiveness and the ego-protective nature of the individual client, quite often there is a great degree of uncertainty in the mind of the therapist as to the reality of the roles which are being reported to him and when it is evident that there is a reality base for some of the reports he receives from an antagonistic spouse, the question remains concerning the impact of this reported role, the substance of the role, and its prevalence. When a marriage starts deteriorating, it is quite natural for each partner to try to justify his position and to displace blame and responsibility for the deterioration of the marriage through recriminations and the imputing of negative roles on the other partner.

Group work is an ideal approach to be used in separating and

3

understanding these diverse roles which are so basic in the marital interaction. As the therapist observes the individuals and their roles within the group he can make a direct connection between the role an individual adopts in the group setting and the one he tends to play most often in the marital setting. In individual counseling, the client may appear somewhat passive, withdrawn, taciturn, and relate his reaction to others and his reaction to events in a philosophical manner. However, in group interactions, it is quite possible for him to change drastically and become the aggressor rather than the passive receptor in a relationship. The following types of behavior are deleterious to a marriage and may be observed in the marriage relationship. We will discuss them as they fall along a continuum from highly aggressive behavior through the acceptance seeker, the sympathy seeker, the confessor, the externalizer, the isolate, the dominator, and the antagonist. Many of these roles will not be exhibited in individual counseling with the marriage partner; however, the group therapist will see them emerge as the group begins to interact.

The Aggressive Individual

As mentioned above, an individual may appear somewhat passive in his relationship to others and his reaction to events may appear as if he is a passive receptor in a relationship. However, when observed in a group setting, it may become obvious that a drastic change has occurred and in reality he is a highly aggressive individual. As an aggressor, he may work many ways to exert his will. He may be oblivious or unconcerned about the feelings of others. He may override their concerns by deflating them, attempting to relegate them to lower status, either expressing disapproval or ignoring their feelings, their value system, or the acts in which they engage and which are counter to his basic goals. He will appear to be highly goal-oriented regardless of the cost in achieving that goal and he will work toward the goal regardless of the hurt feelings, the damage to his interpersonal relationships. He works toward the goal which he perceives as the one bringing him most recognition. Under this set of circumstances, this individual will be most manipulative in that he will show the highest degree of Machiavellianism in the group. He will be somewhat jealous of individuals who gain more recognition than he, and he will be sympathetic toward the individual whom he outshines most readily. Yet this individual may see himself as a somewhat passive person and have little or no understanding of the obvious sources of marital discord.

The Acceptance Seeker

Related to the individual who has a high degree of need to accomplish the goals he perceives as important and who accomplishes them through aggressive-type behavior is the individual whose concern is not the accomplishment of the goals but whose goal is to receive acceptance by the group or one who feels the need for recognition within the group. This is an individual who is quite insecure and tends to need almost continual positive reinforcement as to his self-adequacy and his value to the group or to the marriage partner. This type of individual demonstrates his needs in the group in many ways. Generally, he will not be as oriented toward the goal which is perceived by the group as the group goal as will be the aggressive-type individual. But he will work toward the goal if he feels it will bring a great deal of recognition. Much of his overt behavior upon examination will be seen to be self-serving and self-gratifying behavior rather than goal-oriented behavior. It has been our experience in group work with marriage partners that this type of individual has many more needs than the aggressive-type individual. If the individual who is seeking the recognition to the exclusion of everything else has a spouse who attempts to meet these needs, quite often the needs are so great the spouse loses the impact she once had to fulfill his needs; therefore, he looks elsewhere for the recognition which is so essential to his personality integration. He responds to her as being unconcerned about him, as not really understanding his motivations, and may give the impression that the spouse is somewhat self-centered and uncooperative in the marriage pact. In the group situation, the individual demonstrates his need for recognition by behavior and mannerisms both verbal and nonverbal which call attention to himself. He quite often will boast; he will feel the need to relate personal experiences; he will relate his accomplishments and achievements; perhaps he may relate them in a thinly veiled manner under the guise of using them as an example to make a point in some other area; however, he feels compelled to bring forth his accomplishments, his values, his attributes to the group and to hold them out for group approval. His most painful moments in the group will be when he perceives he has been devalued by other members in the group and placed in an inferior position or when he feels he is demonstrating behavior which is characterized by the group as inadequacy.

The Sympathy Seeker

On a continuum down from the aggressive-type individual on to the individual who is seeking recognition from the group, the next type of personality may be characterized as the sympathy seeker. This individual attempts to elicit responses of sympathy from the group thereby obviating any pressures for him to achieve either within the group or without the group. As he depreciates himself and relegates himself to a lower inferior position, he gets the sympathy of the group and at the same time is absolved of responsibility within the group. This provides him a haven of irresponsibility. He is able to go his own way; he can follow the group or he can elect to remain aloof from the group all with the approval of the group as a result of his being in a position to receive sympathy from the group. As the group becomes more demanding and insistent on his contributing, he will reinforce his protestations of inferiority or illness, of devaluation or of a generalized inadequacy. He will attempt to reinforce the group's feelings of sympathy for him in order to free himself from entanglements of the group. If he is unsuccessful in his attempts to get sympathy from the group, he will attempt to split the group into smaller units and will seek statements of sympathy from the smaller subgroups. The value of the group interaction is to denote how an individual who is a sympathy seeker in the group setting, but who, in the marriage relationship and when seen on an individual counseling basis, may come through as a relatively independent sort of person who expresses feelings of adequacy and concern for the marriage relationship. The group setting will highlight change when his behavior is observed and the pressures of the group are exerted.

The Confessor

The next type of behavior which is brought out in a group is the confessing behavior. This is behavior that is characterized by rather superficial confessing. As the individual sees that the demands are getting greater to reveal himself and as he sees that his responsibility will have to be fulfilled if he is to maintain membership in the group, quite often he starts confessing in a very superficial manner to the group. Generally, these confessions are characterized by large quantity with a very low quality. He feels that the more he confesses, the more he absolves himself of responsibility for honest group interaction. He confesses to his feelings which are somewhat insignificant in a very sober, concerned fashion. He professes to have immediate insight as a result of the group sessions. When an individual starts to criticize him, this confessing-type individual immediately stifles the criticism or stifles the comments by agreeing with the critic and going even further in confessing these feelings or attributes and feelings and attributes related to these on and on *ad nauseam*.

In a marriage, confessing-type behavior is a very effective defense. It is quite frustrating when a marriage partner tries to communicate and is thwarted by the other marriage partner's superficial self-confessing behavior. Communication in this instance is effectively blocked when one marriage partner evades a confrontation with the other marriage partner by this superficial type of confessing behavior. When this type of behavior is exhibited, it is quite difficult to get to the core of the problem in individual counseling since the confessor is verbalizing a great deal of concern, flexibility, and willingness to cooperate when in fact his behavior is aimed more at stifling communication and blocking effective understanding within the marriage relationship. By adopting this defensive behavior, he is not required to engage in a confrontation with the other marriage partner. He is able to maintain interaction on a relatively superficial level.

The Externalizer

Another type of behavior which is exhibited in groups can be characterized by the term "externalization." The externalizer is an individual who becomes uncomfortable in the interaction and the "give and take" which is occurring in the group or which occurs in close interpersonal relationships; he tends to focus on problems that are external to the group or external to the relationship. As the group starts to focus on the individual or as the group gets too close to the individual, he starts externalizing in order to shift the brunt of an attack or the brunt of an inquisition from him on to some external object. Quite often this can be a very effective maneuver; however, again, it is one which is highly frustrating to an individual who is seriously trying to resolve conflicts. An effective externalizer is able to communicate his values, his impressions, his attitudes and beliefs very effectively without referring to himself. He does this through interjecting or projecting his attitudes into the attitudes of groups external to the interaction he is currently engaged in. Consequently, he is able to communicate a point of view which he holds without allowing others to adequately communicate their points of view.

The Isolate

The next type of behavior which is observed in the group setting and has a direct referent back to marital interactions is the isolate. This is the individual who decides to insulate himself from the interaction of the group. He very definitely elects not to interact with the group and decides to disallow the group now interacting with him. He quite often will make a very studied effort to inform the group of his nonchalance, of his decision to be noninvolved. He does this quite often by engaging in stratagems which are distracting to the group but which give no indication of his interest or willingness to contribute to the group. He may attract the attention of one or two other members of the group and start to play with them. He may become very animated in doodling. He may develop little games which he plays with himself such as folding paper, making airplanes, drawing pictures of the room. When confronted, his general response is, "I'm paying attention," "I'm listening," "I'm participating," "I just engage in these little activities to heighten my sensitivity to what's going on." This individual generally will not allow himself to be drawn into the interaction within the group. He will stay outside the mainstream of activity and will attempt to communicate his intentions to stay outside the mainstream of activity through nonverbal behavior. His verbal behavior will be one of conciliation and concern.

The Dominator

The next type of behavior on the continuum from highly goal-oriented to highly negativistic will be the individual who tries to dominate one or more individuals in the group or tries to dominate the entire group. His drives toward domination are an effort to convince others of his authority and of his superiority. His interests are not as goal-oriented as the aggressive-type individual who sacrifices others' feelings and his own interpersonal relationship with others in an effort to accomplish a group goal; however, the dominating-type individual is concerned with exerting influence over others not for the goal which can be achieved but just for the sake of dominance. If there is a highly aggressive individual in the group and a dominating individual in the group, the more maladaptive type of behavior will be exhibited by the dominating individual for he will find the need to express his adequacy by wooing group members away from the goal-oriented aggressive-type individual whose drives are to move the group toward a goal. The dominator will achieve his purpose if he subverts the actions or intents of the aggressive individual. The dominating individual is concerned with achieving a status of respect. He may do this through many types of behavior such as being punitive and using the threat of punitive behavior to tower a weaker member. He may use flattery to woo a member. He may use the power of suggestion and persuasion or he may just attempt to verbally and socially overpower the other individuals to force them into submission. In a marriage relationship, this type individual most often has to have a wife who is somewhat passive and one who does not have a high level of need for individuality and expressions of self-adequacy through the approval of their spouse.

The Antagonist

The next and last type of behavior to be discussed is the antagonist. This is the individual who strives for self-adequacy and recognition through the negativistic behavior and values he adopts. He is somewhat arbitrary and capricious in his value judgments. The underlying constant of his judgments is the contrariness of his position. He seems to be at odds with the mainstream of opinion, values, or actions within the group interaction. His negativism can be quite harsh and sharp. He apparently is unconcerned about the feelings of others in the group. The most important thing to him is to exhibit his individuality by disagreeing with the group consensus. He is stubbornly resistent to coercion or persuasion. He will go so far as to disrupt the flow of the work of the group by attempting to change directions, change the topic of concern, alter the goal which the group is working toward, or try to redefine the ground rules which were established in the group. This antagonist takes a negative view of life and is antagonistic to almost all of the members in the group. He is argumentative and can be quite bombastic when thwarted.

Individual and Group Approaches

There is an exercise in group behavior which requires working toward the solution of a problem concerned with being marooned on the moon. The problem requires individuals to react by rank ordering a number of various types of equipment which they would choose to have with them if they were so marooned. The exercise which has been checked by space experts at the National Space and Aeronautics Administration is first completed by individuals and later by a group of six to eight persons working together. The usual result of the exercise is that group behavior is demonstrated over and over again to be more effective in getting at correct solutions to problems than has individual effort alone. In some few cases the individual's decision may be more effective than that of the group, but in most cases the group decision is more nearly correct than the individual one.

The purpose of the exercise is to demonstrate the effectiveness of group interaction in problem solving. Just as the exercise does demonstrate the effectiveness of increased interaction among individuals in problem solving so does group marital counseling achieve much more in many cases than does the basic interaction between the client and therapist. While much can be accomplished by individual sessions with the client, it is our feeling that supplemental group sessions can bring about enormous strides in understanding and adjustment.

In marital counseling, it is essential to see the clients in an individual one-to-one situation. It is equally important to see spouses together; however, we feel that it is of utmost importance for effective marriage counseling to supplement individual counseling with group techniques, for it is through group techniques that much of the behavior which can remain enigmatic in individual counseling is delineated and exemplified by pressures and interactions of the group. Much of the behavior which has constituted irritant factors of the marriage pact are elicited in the group situation. This type of behavior is on the surface in the group. It can be observed by the therapist and in individual sessions which follow can be related to the individual and interpreted for him to review and evaluate and react to. Without benefit of the group, marital counseling is much slower and a much longer process. Many times, marriage will continue to deteriorate at a faster rate than the therapist is able to diagnose and treat the irritants which are precipitating the deterioration.

Selection of Group Participants

In group marital counseling one generally has a decision to make concerning whether he wants to have in his group only husbands, only wives or mix the group. He also needs to make a decision whether husbands and wives will be in the same group. When husband and wife are in the same group, other members of the group can help them explore in considerable detail their problem areas. When husbands or wives are in groups made up of exclusively all males or all females the group leader will experience some difficulty in keeping the session from turning into a type of complaint session about the opposite sex. When husbands and wives are in groups separately from one another, group members have been shown to be very eager to help the individual to explore his marital situation and understand it more fully. The best combination seems to be one in which both husband and wife are in the same group or husband or wife are in mixed groups of males and females. Heterogeneity has a great affect upon the effectiveness in group interaction and problem solving. Diversity brings with it certain breadth of experience and increases the strength of the group to solve both individual problems and group problems. Persons from all walks of life can be mixed in a heterogeneous marital group counseling situation. This same opinion would extend to persons of various ages and socio-economic backgrounds.

RELATIONSHIPS NECESSARY FOR EFFECTIVE GROUP INTERACTION

Some of the necessary ingredients for effective group problem exploration include acceptance of others, awareness, self acceptance of individuals in the group, and problem centering approaches to behavior. When these conditions exist a high "trust" level has been achieved. People are free to be themselves when a level of trust has been established in the group. When the "trust" level has not been established or is low, group members tend to be manipulative, to hold back information about themselves, and to be defensive. When individuals within the group trust one another defensiveness is reduced, information flow is multiplied, and the strategies of manipulation are dissipated.

The group leader must create in members a feeling of freedom. They can be most valuable as group members to others in groups and themselves when they are free and able to be themselves.

Modeling Behavior

It is the responsibility of the group leader to model the types of behavior which he would like to see exhibited by the various members of the group. The group facilitator or leader should not be overbearing or dominating as a leader but should move the group toward understanding of problems through various behaviors which he not only demonstrates but models. The group leader should be an individual who is friendly, warm, and accepting. He should be a person who works with others and does not practice techniques upon them. The word "with" suggests that the procedure taking place is a relationship and not a technique oriented process. The atmosphere within the group should be productive of or conducive to good mental and social-psychological health. The goal of all group work is that of the obtainment of good mental health.

Every member of the group should be accorded enough consideration and respect by the group in order that he has at least a modicum of self-esteem. The individual must be willing and able to accept himself within a group setting. He must feel that he has the respect of others and that he is a person of worth. The group environment should facilitate the development and maintenance of self-esteem.

Members of the group should show considerable acceptance of others and their attitudes regardless of whether or not group members agree with the attitudes or ideas which are being expressed. In other words, group members do not have to agree with the ideas in order to accept them as legitimate personal feelings of the individual expressing them. At times the needs of individuals in the group for self-esteem may interfere with their accepting and respecting others. It has been shown many times that we may want to feel superior to others and we do this by bolstering ourselves. When this is the case, often the person involved does not have enough respect for himself; therefore, he cannot respect others. Listening to another is the simplest and one of the most basic ways through which we can show respect for him.

Group members need to show understanding of others' feelings and the group leader should demonstrate that he understands how others feel and wishes to get to know them better. If the group leader uses psychological terminology glibly, he may "turn off" the group. He should not attempt to demonstrate understanding through such use of professional jargon, but he should demonstrate that he has what has been called accurate empathy in reference to the individual. He can put himself in the other's place and understand feelings as the other person experiences them.

All members of the group must demonstrate some degree of confidence in the other persons in the group. There must be recognition of the rights and privileges and freedoms to action of others. The group must be characterized by sincerity, integrity, openness, and honesty if it is to achieve its goals. These characteristics help eliminate the threat and help to create an environment in which the individual can develop to his fullest potential by exploring all aspects of his particular marital problem. The group leader should give his attention, respect, understanding, and interest to those within the group who are attempting to work toward a solution of their problems and help others in doing likewise.

Artificiality must be avoided on the part of the group leader at all costs. There is no real alternative to genuineness in the group counseling process.

The group leader must demonstrate the types of behavior which participants in the group need to exhibit if problem solving is to take place. There must be a certain amount of risk taking, in other words, individuals in the group must go beyond what is known to be factual in order to explore their behavior. Persons must be willing to do more than play it safe. If for instance, within a session an individual becomes angry or anxious, these behaviors can make him appear foolish; but these may be necessary behaviors and necessary risks to take in order for him to achieve success in problem solving. There must be substantial support for others as members attempt to reach goals that are important. Persons can say in various ways that they may not be sure what an individual is aiming toward or proposing, but they support the efforts being made to get something moving or to make others understand a particular problem.

There should be a demonstration that persons are free and

able to be open about their feelings and thoughts, and there should be a problem centering or focusing on problems faced by a group rather than on control or method. Problem centering is based upon the assumption that the group can accomplish much more when individuals in groups learn how to solve problems rather than by the leader having to employ certain technique patterns in order to achieve goals. Group members should clearly recognize the feelings of others and how one's feelings are interinfluencing the behavior of others.

Another characteristic which is most important in achieving the level of problem solving ability necessary for success is that of the individual feeling that he can accept his own emotions without denying them or giving rationalizations or apologies. Such acceptance can be evidenced by such statements, "I am disgusted or bored with myself because I feel ineffective."

Problems Which May Surface During Group Marital Counseling

There is no end to the types of human situations which may come to light during marital counseling. Group marital counseling just as individual counseling and other group counseling covers the whole realm of human life and experience. Of course, there are sex problems which include frigidity, sterility, impotence and others. There are the problems of children, there are the problems of incongruencies in expectations, of differences in opinion concerning careers, there is the problem of extramarital relationships, of changing life styles in a rapidly moving society, of parents and in-laws and their influence in the marriage. There are identification problems, problems of personal values, the different meanings of love and substitutes for it which are meaningful to some people and not meaningful to others, the expression and management of feelings, the handling of various financial crises and many others.

The counselor concerned with group marital counseling must be a mature individual who is able to facilitate human learning through the demonstration of the behaviors described earlier. He must know group interactions well and thoroughly understand human behavior.

GROUND RULES FOR GROUP MARITAL SESSIONS

Human interaction includes two major properties: (1) content and (2) process. Content has to do with the subject matter with which the group is concerned. Process has to do with the actual procedure of what is happening between and to group members while the group is working. The group leader must be sensitive to the group process in order to help the group in diagnosing special problems so that these can be dealt with soon and effectively.

One of the important concepts in group interaction is that everyone who is in the group belongs there because he simply is there. Gendlin (1968) has indicated that this concept is one of the most important ones in effecting successful group behavior. If an individual gets angry with another person, this behavior does not change his belonging in the group. If a person reads himself out of a group, it does not change his belonging in it. If he gives up on himself, the group does not give up on him.

Each person determines what is true for him by what is in him according to Gendlin. Whatever he feels makes sense in himself and whatever way he wishes to live inside himself is determined by what is in him as an individual. Most people live mostly inside themselves. No one knows more about how a person really is than the person himself. The group leader should remember that he should force no one to be more honest than he wants to be just at the moment he is speaking. We should listen for the person who is inside the individual who is living and feeling. This person may not be totally exposed to us at any given time although he may wish to be exposed.

The group leader is always responsible for protecting the belongingness of every member to the group and also their right to be heard. He is also responsible for the confidential aspect of the group disclosures, which means that no one will repeat anything which has been said outside of the group unless it concerns only himself.

Everyone should participate in the group. One indication of involvement is verbal participation. The group leader should look for differences in terms of who are the high and low participators. What are the shifts in participation? How are the persons who are not participating being treated by the others? What subgroups are there? Who keeps the group moving? Which of the groups are high in terms of influence? Are there autocrats and peacemakers? Are there members getting attention by their apparent lack of involvement in the group? Who attempts to include everyone in group discussion decision making? In other words, what are the styles of influence? Is the group drifting from topic to topic? Is this a defensive type of behavior? Do they attempt to become overly organized at the expense of losing effectiveness in problem solving? Are there persons outside of the group?

Is the group avoiding certain topics and setting certain norms for behavior? Is religion or sex avoided, for instance, as a topic? Are the group members being overly nice to each other? Are they agreeing too soon, in short are they avoiding facing individual and group problems?

One of the helpful techniques which can be used in group marital counseling is that of spontaneous role playing. This can be done by husband and wife actually sitting in the center of the group and playing out a particular problematic situation. The group members can then react to various aspects of the role playing and make suggestions in order that the individuals may develop fuller understanding of the problem area. It may also be useful to have a surrogate wife or husband role play with an actual husband or wife.

Role reversal is another technique in which individuals reverse their roles and then role play actual situations. This technique can be most interesting in that the husband plays the wife's part and wife plays the husband's part. It is sometimes easy to bring about understanding through the use of this technique. Persons can relive past events or project future occurrences through role playing.

Another technique which is useful is that of repeating the client's key words or statements. This is particularly useful in terms of what has been called free association. In other words, that process of using clues or cues to help the client give meaningful information about himself and his problems.

The group leader should keep in mind that persons who live many psychosomatic complaints may be disguising personal problems and conflicts. He should also remember that the individual group member who offers any complaints about his spouse may be covering his own personal anxieties and inadequacies.

TIME PERIODS AND TYPES OF SESSIONS

The purpose of this chapter has been to describe group marital counseling. Generally, sessions may last for three to four hours and may be ongoing meeting eight to ten or more times. This varies from the individual counseling sessions which usually last from 50 to 60 minutes.

Much of the material given in this chapter concerns the facilitating of groups rather than the actual leading of them as a group therapist. It is felt by the authors that selected encounter group concepts can be of substantial benefit in various types of marital counseling.

Of course, it may be that group members will wish to engage in a type of marathon encounter in which they may continue their group activities for 20-24 hours. These sessions can later be followed by shorter two to three hour sessions of follow-up groups for those who are interested. Group leaders should not become discouraged if some of their group members do not choose to return to later group meetings. People vary enormously in their abilities to withstand various types of stress and many people feel a good deal of insecurity and stress during group counseling work even though substantial efforts have been made to establish an atmosphere of warmth and trust. Some people are able to gain a great deal in a short period of time and for these persons, individual counseling may be more in accordance with their needs than group experiences.

The group counselor, leader, or facilitator—whichever name is chosen—must keep in mind that the purpose of the session is whatever goal the group decides upon. At times a group session may provide real service in terms of being informational in nature. One of the basic problems related to problems in marriage is the preparation for simply living with another person.

At times the counselor will find it necessary to assume the role of information giver and tutor in individual sessions and in group sessions when members find it necessary to be informational in order to achieve basic goals which have been established. Group members can greatly help individuals in the group by exploring the needs of each person. In many cases unmet needs exist due to the fact that these needs are not understood by the spouse and often the person himself.

REFERENCE

Gendlin, E. T., and Beebe, J.: Experiential groups: Instructions for groups. In Gazda, G. M. (Ed.): *Innovations to Group Psychotherapy.* Springfield, Ill.: Charles C Thomas, 1968, pp. 190-206.

Chapter II

FAMILIES IN CRISIS

Gilbert L. Ingram

■ Historical Perspective on the Family
■ The Family and Delinquency
■ Working With the Family in Crisis
■ The Future

The family as a viable social unit is under attack from many different sources in modern American society. The assaults have increased in both intensity and number, ranging from criticism concerning the family's lack of effectiveness in producing adaptable members of society, to demands for elimination of the family as it is presently constituted (Cooper, 1970). An immediate result of these assaults is exemplified in the present chapter; many researchers and practitioners are being compelled to look closely at what is happening.

The spectacle is depressing and indeed presents a sad commentary on the family's efficacy as a social unit. Because 50 percent of delinquents come from broken homes, the fact that families are increasingly being broken by desertion and divorce is of immediate concern. Of those units that manage to remain intact, the adult family members manifest their social and emotional problems in various ways, such as alcoholism, drug addiction, crime, and suicide. These problems naturally extend to children of the unhappy families.

Past dissatisfactions of observers toward the family generally were aimed at the lower class of society and thus were more easily dismissed as problems peculiar to that segment of the population. Today, the delinquent products of inadequate, unstable family units are visible in every social class and cannot be ignored so easily.

Theorists and practitioners of diverse persuasions seem to agree that the family is of fundamental importance in the occurrence of delinquency. Every involved discipline, despite differences in emphasis, joins in the general castigation of the family. Typical of these views are the following: "It is a truism that for every juvenile delinquent, there is a delinquent home environment. Children are not born delinquent; they are made that way by their families, usually by their parents" (CRM's *Developmental Psychology Today*, 1971, p. 291). "The more thorough a study of juvenile delinquency is, the greater the emphasis laid on the family as a social unit" (Pettit, 1970, p. 191).

The family is frequently cited as the villain of many social evils but with regard to delinquency there is almost unanimous agreement. Even in those cases in which other economic, cultural and psychological factors play a major role, the family still remains significant by its failure to counteract these other forces.

Research results notwithstanding, it is possible that this consensus is nothing more than an empty generalization, devoid of any real meaning and worthless for purposes of prevention or treatment. In fact, such a broad indictment of the family may seduce some into thinking that they now understand the problem, when obviously, this is not the case.

Another fallacy in this area is the tendency to use preliminary research results to place a label on a family that seems to breed delinquency. Once this label is available, the assumption is made that a grasp on the cause of delinquency is at hand. Hypostatization is a comforting but nonproductive enterprise. The causes of delinquency are undoubtedly complex and varied, and not unitary.

It is not the intention to present a comprehensive review of all literature pertaining to the effect of the family on delinquent behavior. This task, although necessary, has been accomplished by others, including an excellent review by Peterson and

Becker (1965). Rather, the goal is an overview of the area emphasizing general conclusions that appear to have some merit and more importantly, that may have some applicability. Problems in working with the families of delinquents are discussed and specific examples of tactics are presented that may facilitate successful intervention.

HISTORICAL PERSPECTIVE ON THE FAMILY

The modern concept of childhood was unknown in the Middle Ages. At that time, childhood was viewed exclusively as a transition stage before adulthood. As the rate of infant mortality and the demand for productive work decreased, the family began to focus on the child as an individual in his own right. Children were able to go to school and refrain from work. Especially during the 17th and 18th Centuries with the increased opportunity for education, childhood assumed the status of a separate stage of development. Adolescence as a separate stage was even later in evolving, not appearing in its present state until the late 19th and early 20th Centuries.

During most of the 19th Century, the agrarian-based culture predominated with its independent family unity and a cohesive community life. As the industrial culture grew, family structure loosened with the concentration of populations in the large, heterogeneous communities. The shift was not only rural to urban, but also included an increased immigration from Europe to the big cities of this country. It should be noted that separate courts for juveniles were first established in the late 19th Century after the large metropolitan courts were swamped with an increasing number of juvenile offenders.

Long cited as a puzzling and difficult stage, adolescence gained society's concentrated attention after the late 19th Century. Because of the rapid technological advances and the influence of mass media, the present situation provides even more stress for the teenager and the family. As Mead aptly stated, "Parents have been rearing unknown children for an unknown world since about 1946" (Mead, 1972, p. 586).

Added to the ordinary pains and adaptations that occur in

growing up during any historical period, today's teenager is placed in various conflict situations. While being bombarded with provocative stimuli and the sight of hedonistic behaviors of adults, the adolescent is taught to remain economically unproductive and to postpone immediate satisfaction for long range goals. Yet, after a prolonged period of protection and abstinence from "adult" activities, he is supposed to emerge somehow from this dependent status into adulthood fully capable of behaving in a responsible manner. Added to these contradictory messages, which confuse and frustrate most adolescents, are the other social changes that have altered family life.

The size of the typical family has decreased so that each member is interacting with fewer other members, making individual contributions all the more important. At the same time, shared family activity or "togetherness" has diminished, and this restricts the number of intrafamilial interactions. This trend sometimes prevents the family's carrying out its prescribed social function. The once biological contribution of the family was that of providing economic and physical safety for the members. Today, society expects the family to serve primarily as a socialization mechanism for the child and to provide satisfaction of psychological needs for all family members.

Leadership of the family has shifted in many ways from a patriarchal type to a more democratic or shared method of decision making. The former role of the father, that of providing explicit authority and fulfilling visible economic duties, allowed the children to model after him. He was quickly accepted as the authority figure. The mother's role was also definite and visible. Changing roles plus the extensive impact of mass media have created a situation in which children are less likely to accept the parents as models of behavior. Riesman (1969) has written of the increasing separatism of teenage culture and the massing in schools of large numbers of young people. The atmosphere engendered by this phenomenon is one of questioning the legitimacy of adult authority. In fact, Riesman believes that the young become "captives" of each other.

The shift in parental roles also has direct effects on the child when problems occur between the parents. One immediate result is seen in the handling of child custody cases. Until recently, fathers were considered to own all family property, including the children. The mother for all practical purposes had no legal rights to them. Today, an almost automatic preference obtains for the mother over the father in such court decisions.

Another characteristic of modern families is their increased mobility. Many writers describe the family as completely inefficient social units, citing the nomadic nature of their existence and resultant lack of stability. All of these modern trends in the life style of family units have dramatic effects on the children. The smaller size of the family plus the frequent changes in residence creates a lack of personal ties with others. Most modern families work and recreate as separate individuals outside of their home neighborhood. It is no great surprise that children of such families feel alienated, disenchanted, and at odds with the world around them.

Granted that modern families have unique problems and do not seem to be satisfying society's expectations; why though do seemingly privileged teenagers become delinquent, especially in terms of violent acting-out behavior? The attribution of such behavior to lower-class versus middle-class persons had been accepted as a general belief in both lay and professional circles. More recently, Stark and McEvoy (1972) among others have challenged this assumption. Using data compiled by the National Commission on the Causes and Prevention of Violence, they cited statistics supporting the idea that, in fact, the middle class is more prone toward physical assault than the poor. Stark and McEvoy suggested that violence among the poor is more likely to become a police matter because of lack of privacy and little recourse to professional counselors or influential friends.

Keniston (1968) has cited one reason for some of the problems of modern families that offers a different perspective on violence. The adolescent's constant exposure to social upheavals occurring during the past decades has afforded an excellent opportunity for disagreeing with parental values and for perceiving the discrepancy between what parents say and what they do.

Keniston acknowledges that there has always been a failure to live up to professed ideals, but heretofore the adolescent has learned when parents can be reasonably expected to practice what they preach. Today, this "institutionalization of hypocrisy" does not occur so easily because rapid social change does not allow for the easy definition of exceptions to the rule and it is much easier for youth to detect such discrepancies. Ironically, the young hold to those values (love of fellow man, equality for all) which their parents espouse but do not practice. Having been raised in an affluent environment, the adolescent feels outrage over the lack of opportunities for those less fortunate. Added to this general feeling of anger and disappointment with his parents is the ever-present fear caused by the threat of the bomb and possible technological death. The awareness of violence is continually reinforced by frequently publicized mob behaviors.

Whether the cause is frustration over living conditions, personal inadequacies, or as Keniston has suggested, an obsession concerning violence in general, there is little doubt that the tendency to act out antisocially is increasing among youth in all social classes.

Today, if the family were considered to be a small business enterprise, it might have to declare bankruptcy. The task of turning out a useful social product is not being accomplished. In a recent large-scale study, the authors concluded that most teenagers do not achieve emotional autonomy, detachment from the family, or a personal ethical code of behavior (Douvan and Adelson, 1966). Although these manifestations of inadequate families are possibly as significant as delinquency, none produce such immediate and tangible damage against society. While the financial cost of delinquency is astronomical by all estimates, the psychological and sociological effects are undoubtedly a greater liability for everyone.

THE FAMILY AND DELINQUENCY

Numerous studies have been conducted in the investigation of family characteristics and delinquent behavior. Too many of these studies suffer from severe methodological weaknesses. The typical strategy used in those studies that seem to satisfy research requirements has been a comparison of families of delinquents with families of nondelinquents. This shotgun approach has been necessary because no systematic theory is available to guide inquiry and to organize existing data. The growing emphasis on differential classification programs and the concomitant development of differential treatment approaches acknowledge what every practitioner knows; i.e., delinquents do not present themselves as a homogeneous group for research or treatment purposes. Similarly, families of delinquents have their own particular "personality" and do not as a single group share similar characteristics.

Rubenfeld (1967) identified the lack of a framework for family classification as a serious drawback in any attempt to determine the effect of family life on delinquent behavior. However, his suggestion for categorizing families by use of child-rearing patterns, such as those determined by the Fels Institute, may also be a waste of time. For example, after reviewing the enormous amount of data on the effect of different child-rearing practices, McCandless (1967) presented his advice which seems most appropriate: ". . . mothers [parents] who are well-meaning and who try relaxedly to do what they sincerely believe is best for their children—particularly when this is in harmony with the cultural ways of the community with which they are most closely associated—obtain the best results with their children" (McCandless, 1967, pgs. 127-128). We have little reliable data on the subject considering the widely scattered attention directed toward it.

Despite the lack of information concerning the family, research findings have indicated possible characteristics that may bear on the problem. Three general types of families have consistently been identified with delinquent behavior: an unhappy, disrupted home with poor structure; a home in which parental attitudes of rejection prevail, and; homes demonstrating a lack of consistent and adequate discipline. Whenever possible, representative studies from both the earlier and the more current literature are presented.

Disrupted Homes and Delinquency

Families may be disrupted by the physical loss of a member through death, divorce, or separation, or by the lack of structure caused by disturbed or criminalistic parents. Many studies in this area have been devoted to the effect of father absence on delinquent males, but the investigation of that variable has been a recent phenomenon.

A widely held assumption had been that the mother produced the major effect on the children and the father was relatively unimportant. Freud's writings were largely responsible for this focus on the mother's role, and even his critics seemed to agree with him on this one issue. The effect of maternal deprivation dominated the literature for many years. However, as more interest developed concerning the father's role, studies began to demonstrate the influence of the father, particularly concerning delinquency. Glueck and Glueck (1962) cited repeated instances of alcoholism, nonsupport, brutality, and frequent absence from home in the fathers of delinquent boys. Extreme difficulties with male authority figures were frequently noted (see Medinnus, 1965) but disturbed relations with mothers were present only for a few delinquents (Brigham, Rickets, & Johnson, 1967).

As attention was directed more toward the father, new problems were encountered which interfered with research. If the family is intact, fathers usually work during the day and have to be contacted in evenings or on weekends. Because this involvement entails the loss of leisure time, fathers are less likely to cooperate. Fathers also view themselves as having little to do with their children's problems because they share the same cultural bias that others have. If the father is unavailable, researchers have frequently adopted another approach which has severe limitations; namely, interviews are held with the mother to obtain information about the father. Distorted perceptions are typically obtained, either positively biased when the home is intact or negatively biased when the home is broken. Both kinds of distortions interfere with comparisons of fatherless homes and intact homes.

Available data from those studies that have been conducted on the effect of fatherless homes indicate that the way in which the father leaves the family is an important variable. For example, loss of either parent through death does not seem to be as harmful an experience as a separation because of parental discord.

When the father is absent from the home, the effect apparently centers on disturbed social behaviors for boys. Father absence produced poor sex typing (Bach, 1946) and poor social relations (Stolz, 1954). Because these factors have been associated with delinquency, the effect of father absence on delinquent behavior seems quite important. The question of the relation of the child's age when father absence occurs to subsequent delinquent behavior is another issue far from being settled. Lynn and Sawrey (1959) and Siegman (1966) found that father absence before age five often produced compensatory masculine behavior in adolescence. More recently, Biller (1971) reviewed the literature and concluded that absence during the elementary school years was most important for the development of delinquency.

The importance of father absence for delinquency is not limited to lower class children. Siegman (1966) asked a group of medical students anonymously to reveal their early histories. Minor behavior problems such as cheating in school were equally likely to occur in both father-absent and father-present groups, but serious acts such as theft of property occurred more frequently in the father-absent group.

Recognizing the importance of a variable and isolating its particular effect are two entirely different problems. Although many studies do support the notion that fatherless homes frequently result in delinquency, approaching the problem simply in terms of father-absence versus intact homes has yielded no definitive answers. Hertzog and Studia (1968) reviewed 59 studies dealing with the effects of fatherlessness on children in general and 13 studies dealing directly with delinquency. They found general support for a relationship between delinquency and fatherless homes but also noted qualifying factors. Their suggestions for future research included a shift from single variable analysis to a study of interacting clusters of factors. The fact that approximately six million children in the United States are being raised in fatherless homes indicates the urgency of proceeding with definitive studies.

Contrary to earlier writings, absence of the mother is not frequently cited as a major factor in the area of delinquency. Most researchers apparently agree with Becker, Peterson, Hellmer, Shoemaker, and Quay (1959) who reported the role of the father as being apparently more important than that of the mother in the development of delinquent behavior. More recently, as the role of the mother has shifted in our society, some attention has been directed toward the possible influence of working mothers on children. However, most studies indicate that that type of temporary absence is not a significant factor.

Emotional disturbance on the part of either parent, which also produces a lack of structure in the home, seems to be instrumental in producing disturbed delinquents. Delinquents who are regarded as emotionally disturbed often have disturbed parents (Becker, et al., 1959; Liverant, 1959; Peterson, Becker, Hellmer, Shoemaker, & Quay, 1959; Richardson & Roebuck, 1965). Many practitioners have discovered that delinquents have character-disordered parents when they attempted unsuccessfully to work with them (Reiner & Kaufman, 1959). The presence of disturbed or criminalistic parents does not distinguish delinquents from other groups, but it does indicate that homes disrupted by disturbed as well as absent parental figures may indeed contribute to antisocial behavior.

Homes may also be disrupted by the lack of physical space and by the chaotic life style that accompanies such an environment. These characteristics typically describe the lower-class family, but as already stated, lack of structure is not confined to the physical aspects of the home. In this sense, middle-class children also are often exposed to a living style that precludes a stable pattern of existence. One immediate result of such disrupted homelife for children from all social classes is to make them more vulnerable to the influence of antisocial peer groups (Peterson & Becker, 1965).

The specific ways in which broken and disrupted homes contribute substantially to the delinquency problem are just beginning to be identified. For example, Wood, Wilson, Jessor, & Bogan (1966) found that the overwhelming feelings of powerlessness that delinquents have in dealing with society can be attributed partly to the lack of meaningful structure in their family life. As yet, few research findings in this area have been substantiated and none have been shown to offer meaningful ideas for application in the real world.

Parental Rejection and Delinquency

Rejection of the child by either or both parents has long been cited as one important factor in aggressive behavior by numerous researchers. For instance, Updegraff (1939), in reviewing the literature concerning the influence of parental attitudes upon the child's behavior, found a positive relation between maternal rejection and overt aggression in the child. Similarly, Baldwin, Kalhorn, and Breese (1945), using data from the Fels project, found that rejected children showed a marked tendency toward quarreling, increased resistance toward adults, and sibling hostility. Bandura and Walters (1959) and Andry (1960) found rejection by the father to be a significant pattern for their delinquent samples. McCord, McCord, and Howard (1961) conducted an extensive study involving direct observations of behavior for more than five years. One of their relevant findings was that parents who generally rejected their sons were most likely to produce aggressive boys. More recently, McCord, McCord, and Howard (1963) suggested that antisocial aggression depends more on the degree of rejection and other parental behaviors than simply the absence or presence of parental rejection.

A great deal more has been written about the effect of parental rejection on a particular type of delinquent or criminal, namely the psychopath. This cruel, defiant person who personifies the laymen's stereotype for all delinquents deserves some special attention because he exhibits extreme variations of behavior found in many delinquents.

Lipman (1951) presented a view which may be taken as a general orientation. He said that the psychopathic child is one who has been rejected from the beginning. Subsequent aggression is almost a compulsive act and no feeling for other people is present. Bender (1961) stated that psychopathic behavior occurs when the child is exposed to early and severe emotional and social deprivation attributable either to impersonal institutional care or to critical blocks in the mother-child relationship. Fox (1961) proposed that the psychopath's lack of internalization of cultural values could result from his unfortunate first contact with society, i.e. extreme rejection by the parents.

This has an interesting analogy in research conducted on animals. Harlow (1962) found that monkeys raised in isolation had severe social abnormalities that could be compared to psychopathic behavior. Among other types of behavior, they showed exaggerated aggression and an absence of affectional interaction. This seems to indicate that the influence of early social relationships on aggressive behavior may hold despite species differences.

Psychopathic behavior has been proposed to stem from parent-child relationships other than extreme rejection. Greenacre (1945) reported the fathers of psychopaths to be usually men who spend little time at home and who act in a cold manner toward the child. The mother was not a steady parent in her interactions with the child or with others. Jenkins (1960) proposed, in addition to the possibility of organic involvement, that the child may have been exposed to a confusing situation for social training. All of these proposals are generally in agreement with the research cited above. Despite the *post facto* nature of the writings, they point to a rejecting environment early in life as a causal factor in aggressive behavior and possibly in the etiology of psychopathy.

Parental Control Techniques and Delinquency

There are three general ways in which parental reactions seem to contribute to delinquency: (1) Parental attempts at discipline are inadequate to control antisocial behavior; (2) Parental reactions provide a punitive model for the child to imitate; and (3)

The parents deliberately encourage the child's inappropriate behavior.

The inadequacy of parental discipline in controlling the delinquent's behavior has been noted by many researchers. Healy and Bronner (1926) and Burt (1929) noted that defective parental discipline was an important social determinant of delinquent behavior. Merrill (1947) determined that most of her delinquents came from homes with lax, erratic, or overly strict discipline. Glueck and Glueck (1950) found that the delinquent's parents, particularly the father, had the same difficulty with discipline. Bandura and Walters (1959), Bennett (1960), and McCord, et al. (1961) cited the inconsistent handling of problem behavior by parents as a factor in delinquency.

The effect of inadequate discipline is hypothesized by Hoffman and Saltzstein (1967) to be the weak development of conscience frequently found in delinquents. Apparently the type of discipline exerted by the parents does not facilitate the increased resistance to temptation which is necessary to prevent antisocial acts.

The second way in which parental control techniques may lead to delinquency is by providing an aggressive model for the child. Bandura, Ross, and Ross (1961, 1963) found that children, especially boys, are influenced by viewing aggressive behavior, and more importantly, become more aggressive themselves in other situations. The significance of these studies is magnified by the fact that parents of delinquents resort more often to aggressive behavior for punishment than do other parents (Glueck & Glueck, 1950; McCord, et al., 1961).

Physical punishment may effectively suppress behavior for a short period but it frequently causes a great deal of frustration and provides another opportunity for the delinquent to learn to be aggressive. As Sears, Maccoby, and Levin (1957) found in their classic study, the pattern of child-rearing that produces the most aggressive children is when the parents disapprove of aggression but punish its occurrence with their own physical aggression or threats of aggression.

The third, and perhaps most insidious manner by which parents may influence the expression of delinquency, is the deliberate encouragement of antisocial acts. A great deal of data has been collected which supports the hypothesis that delinquent behavior is reinforced by the family. Shaw and McKay (1942) and Glueck and Glueck (1950) both found that their delinquents came from homes in which other criminals were living. McCord and McCord (1958) discovered that a criminal father plus the absence of maternal warmth was the one combination most likely to lead to delinquent behavior. Similarly, dropping out of school, which typically accompanies delinquency, is related to the parents exhibiting the same behavior (Williams, 1963).

The above examples of general reinforcement of delinquency are overshadowed by the occurrences of direct antisocial instruction by the parents. Bandura and Walters (1959) noted that parents of aggressive boys tended to encourage aggression. Bandura (1960) found that mothers of aggressive boys were punitive when aggression was expressed toward them but became more tolerant when the aggression was expressed toward peers or siblings. Becker, Peterson, Luria, Shoemaker, and Hellmer (1962) reported that mothers who frequently used physical punishment also frequently told their children to fight other children whenever necessary.

WORKING WITH THE FAMILY IN CRISIS

Although increasing evidence indicates that families are doing a poor job of rearing children, one conclusion remains inevitable under our present system of justice; the family can not be ignored in either the prevention or treatment of delinquents.

In reviewing the history of the development of juvenile courts in this country, Mennel (1972) concluded:

> Today, as then, we can no longer disquality parents from caring for their children simply because they are poor or unfamiliar with the principles of child psychology. Parents may indeed abuse or fail to exercise their disciplinary authority. There is, however, little historical evidence to indicate that public authorities in the United States have provided viable and humane alternatives [p. 78].

Until realistic alternatives are available or society changes its viewpoints regarding the sacrosanctity of the family, involvement of the family is necessary. Even after the delinquent's behavior has become completely unmanageable, the situation in which he does not have to return to his basic family unit would be the rare exception. Unfortunately, even in this case or after incarceration has been effected, the courts have no legal authority to insist upon the parent's involvement in the treatment of the child.

Experience to date indicates that successfully involving the family in the prevention or treatment of delinquency often is dependent upon the individual expertise and initiative of the change agent in overcoming bureaucratic inertia. Few specific suggestions are available from the research literature. However, a full understanding of many of the problems facing the family in crisis better prepares the worker to facilitate this involvement. Several parental reactions to delinquency occur frequently enough to warrant some attention. These reactions include a denial of blame with subsequent anger directed toward society, guilt after the fact and a feeling of helplessness, and finally, passivity and a relinquishing of responsibility because it is now out of their hands.

The Hostile Family

Many families confronted with the fact of their child's delinquency react very negatively. Typically, these are multi-problem families for whom delinquency poses an additional crisis. Already overwhelmed with financial and social misfortunes, the family is ill-prepared to deal realistically with the child's situation. Most hostile families fall into society's lower social classes.

Previous interactions between family members and society's representatives usually have been in relation to problems in the educational system and frequently have been negative experiences. Against this background, the appearance of another "helper" in the life of the family may be greeted with anger and sometimes overt hostility. Communication often breaks down because of real differences which exist between the values and language of the worker and the family.

Not only do the disadvantaged have their own particular vo-

cabulary and style of speech but their concerns in life may differ significantly from the middle-class culture (Miller, 1958).
Typical middle-class workers, regardless of discipline, probably
share common beliefs about human nature (Dole & Nottingham,
1969). Frequently, the workers' beliefs conflict with the family's
own values and communication channels break down. For example, the middle-class emphases on frugality and responsibility
probably are not shared by disadvantaged families. Similarly, the
family may seem unconcerned with long-term plans because
their energies are focused on present problems. Confronted with
an unwelcome stranger who talks differently and places a high
value on the "wrong" things, family members may directly indicate their disagreement and displeasure. Any helper, finding his
well-intentioned overtures to be greeted thusly, can fall into the
trap of assuming an authoritative posture and a condescending
manner. The interaction undoubtedly will proceed downhill
from this point.

What can be done to work with such a family? The answer depends upon the ability of the helper to understand and accept
the members for what they are. This means that he must enter-
tain the idea that the family's behaviors and values may be appropriate *for them*. If he can do that, he should aim at the fa-
cilitation of the child's adaptation by working with the family.
This process entails his gaining acceptance not as a friend but
as someone who can help. Learning the language and values of
the family are important because it is the rare middle-class person who fully appreciates the social and personal lives of the
lower-class individual. Other suggestions that may be of some
use include the following:

1. Any indications of talking down to the family will reinforce their dislike and distrust of the authority person.
2. Refusing to state opinions or backing down when confronted by the family will be interpreted as a sign of weakness and interfere with rapport.
3. Avoidance of some relevant issues for the sake of "being
   nice" will destroy any respect for the person.
4. Firmness, not coldness, is the preferred approach.

5. Programs and suggestions should be geared to the real concerns of the family and not for abstract goals.
6. Giving the family concrete tools to work with is better than speaking in generalities.
7. Providing the family with tangible services, if at all possible, will facilitate their cooperation.
8. Do not expect appreciation, at least in the traditional sense, for these efforts.

Most of these suggestions are self-explanatory. Providing concrete suggestions (#6 above) is discussed in the next session. An example of a tangible service (#7 above) may be the worker's serving as a go-between for the family and the school.

After the disadvantaged child has experienced difficulties in school, attempts by either the teacher or the parent to intervene are usually viewed as interference by the other party. An increasingly negative series of communications may convince the family, for example, that the teacher is either not concerned or is discriminating unfairly against the child. Subsequent school difficulties may be excused by the parents in such an atmosphere of distrust. Serving as a go-between in this case, the worker can make a valuable contribution by soliciting information from the school and by sharing helpful family data with the teacher. One result of such activities may be to discover that the child, accidently or deliberately, has reinforced erroneous assumptions on the part of both teacher and parents. Regardless of the specifics, however, all parties benefit from this type of interchange which minimizes the defensive maneuverings of all concerned.

The best intentions will not always guarantee success in working with the family, especially one predisposed to suspicion and hostility toward outsiders. The practitioner may well find that his contributions are either not accepted or are of limited usefulness. This outcome should suggest another immediate alternative which has proven effective in many instances, namely the use of the community volunteer.

Initial reluctance to use volunteers was a natural reaction from professionals who felt that they and only they could understand and deal with delinquents and their families. However, with the failure of traditional therapy approaches and the scarcity of professionals, the use of lay counselors or family workers has gained in popularity. Using volunteers does not remove the responsibility from the worker. Rather, the professional becomes a case manager at a different level; for example, selection, assignment and training of volunteers is essential for the success of a volunteer program. If done correctly, the use of volunteers can be effective even in the most difficult situations. Carkhuff (1971) has described a successful program to train lay counselors indigenous to the inner city, typically regarded as one of the most resistive areas to reach with any services.

The Inadequate Family

One frequently finds families that want to cooperate but seem incapable of handling their children or at least have difficulty with one particular child. Sometimes the family has reared several children without delinquent histories but another child has run into numerous difficulties. This child may be a special child in that he has been sickly, retarded, brain damaged, left alone for a period because of unavoidable environmental circumstances, or for one reason or another has been afforded special status in the parent's eyes. The inappropriate handling of such a child may lead to delinquency in any social class. Patterson, Cobb, and Ray (1970) found that the types of processes in the family leading to delinquent behavior were present in all socioeconomic levels.

Assuming that the family does want to help their child or that the worker has prepared them for such involvement, the task of the practitioner is to deliver as quickly as possible to the parents techniques for making successful changes in the child's behavior. For reasons both of efficacy and efficiency, behavioral techniques seem to be the treatment of choice. They are the easiest to communicate, easiest to understand, and have been applied successfully with parents in diverse situations. Using the family itself as an agent of social change allows them to assume primary responsibility for the child which enhances feelings of competence and mastery over their environment. Additionally, the techniques are already being used by the parents but typically in an unsystematic fashion. Minuchin, Montalvo, Guerney, Rosman, and Schmer (1967) discovered that the mothers of problem children in slum areas used reinforcement techniques, but inconsistently and inappropriately for the child's deviant behavior.

Some direct results of inappropriate reinforcement techniques on delinquents have been identified. Delinquents, in comparison to nondelinquents, are raised in homes where dependency behavior, approval seeking, and verbalizations of dependent behavior are negatively reinforced (Bandura & Walters, 1959; Bender, 1947; McCord & McCord, 1956). The implications of this extinction of dependency behavior for verbal counseling approaches may explain in part the fact that delinquents do not typically profit from conventional therapy. In fact, Mueller (1969) found that client's behaviors with therapists became increasingly similar to behaviors that occurred within the family constellation.

The strategy of retraining parents to act as more effective behavior modifiers has been successfully applied to parents of disturbed children (see Hirsch & Walder, 1969). The basic idea of using parents as the primary change agents is not only more economical and practical, but Patterson, et al. (1970) cited evidence suggesting that it may have a more permanent effect. Their program, in contrast with other attempts, concentrated on changing multiple classes of deviant child behaviors rather than altering a single behavior. Some of their specific techniques and findings have wider applicability for working with parents than their particular study. Relevant suggestions from their program are summarized below.

1. Having parents simply read programmed texts on child management techniques is of limited value. [As adjunct material, these books may be helpful: *Child Management*, Smith & Smith, 1966; *Living with Children*, Patterson & Gullion, 1968.]

2. Telling parents what to do is not as effective as the actual demonstration of recommended procedures.

3. Training of the parent in the home has the advantage of the normal setting but it is a costly procedure. Group training methods are more advantageous once the family becomes involved in the process.

4. Parents are notoriously inaccurate in remembering their children's early behaviors. Dependable information should be obtained through ongoing recording.

5. Structuring of home visits is necessary to get an adequate observation of the home. Family members often attempt to avoid the "intruder" by remaining in an inaccessible location such as the bedroom. It may be necessary to specify requirements of who is to be present and where during these visits.

6. Observing the behavior of the delinquent by himself is less reliable than watching the behavior of all family members for a period of time.

7. The verbal behavior of parents (everything is fine now; yes, we understand the problem, etc.) should not be accepted at face value without additional evidence of changes in behavior.

8. Providing concrete examples of how to apply behavior principles to everyday problems is more easily understood by parents than the supplying of textbook answers.

9. It may be necessary to become a nuisance to the father in order to obtain his cooperation; i.e. contact him daily, have court personnel call him, etc. The worker should keep in mind that the uncooperative father may be unable to carry out his assigned tasks rather than being deliberately resistive.

10. The parent's starting with a simple behavioral problem between himself and the child maximizes the probability of a successful experience with the techniques.

11. One goal of family training is to teach the parents to intercede before the child's behavior becomes extreme and before physical measures are necessary to control it.

12. Parents should be reassured that an improvement in the behavior of one child does not mean that another child

will increase his deviant behavior. Many parents believe this to be true and sometimes are reluctant to initiate change.

The Family of the Incarcerated Delinquent

After delinquency has progressed to the point requiring institutionalization, it is exceedingly difficult to involve the family in rehabilitation of the delinquent. In addition to the predisposing circumstances which may have existed in the family for some time, the incarceration of the child creates additional problems for the family. Many families react very negatively to the institutionalization, preferring to act as if the problem no longer belongs to them. Others use the physical separation as an excuse to justify feelings of rejection that may have originally contributed to the delinquency. Regardless of the underlying factors, it is imperative that staff members attempt to overcome this obstacle to rehabilitation.

Staff time is not sufficient to allow for home visitation, not to mention the expense involved in such activities. Encouraging the family to meet with staff on institutional visiting days has not proven successful. Unless the family is able to afford weekday trips, which would be most unusual, visits mean weekend hours and the resultant absence of key staff members. Moreover, even when all parties are present, family involvement through visits is not regular enough for meaningful interactions to occur. All of these factors add to the communication gaps and lead to misconceptions for both staff and family. The delinquent suffers directly from the lack of family involvement because parental planning is crucial for release programming but more importantly, because the parent's behavior often has been a contributing factor to the delinquent's present situation.

One recent suggestion has been to invite groups of parents of delinquents to the institution for week long visits (Stollery, 1970). Teams of staff counselors evaluate the delinquent's behavior and plan a unified program for him in conjunction with all family members. This program has the added advantage for low income families of providing a type of family vacation as contrasted with the brief, intermittent visits which may serve as a financial punishment. When groups of parents visit at the same time, it serves to facilitate a sharing of mutual concerns between families. Relaxed communications within the family are stimulated by the structured recreation time and reinforced through the group discussions. Staff as well as family members gain by the family's appreciation for the child's situation, especially pertaining to institutional procedures. Although there are numerous problems inherent in such a program, the results suggest a need for additional innovative attempts along these same lines.

One possible outcome of this type of visitation program may be the family's realization that they are unable to provide the necessary controls for the child. This conclusion is often at odds with their wish for him to remain in the family. After the family accepts their own limitations, they should be much more open to suggestions for new approaches. In this case, for example, a day-care program such as the one described by Post, Hicks, and Monfort (1968) may be appropriate. The child is kept in the home which avoids the guilt or other feelings accompanying removal. However, during the day the child is engaged in a program at a community center which also allows further work with the family. This type of program is less expensive than institutionalization but is more structured than total release to the family setting.

Another possible finding of family evaluation may be that the child cannot be helped by his own family. If the needs of the child cannot be met within the natural family, a foster family may serve the purpose. Witherspoon (1966) described the advantages of foster home placements for juvenile delinquents, particularly when removal of the child from the home community is necessary to interrupt the established chain of delinquency. Special training is of course important for the foster parents as well as counseling to prepare the family to relinquish their legal claims to the child.

Both of the above programs provide alternative modes of action which may be necessary in compensating for some family deficiencies.

THE FUTURE

Despite the growing number of attacks on the family, it probably will continue to exist in its present form for some years. Rather than attacking the family with no productive goals in view, society's energies should be invested in researching the family's effects on delinquency and in modifying existing weaknesses with available resources.

Developing typological approaches to delinquency along dimensions other than social class has proven to be a promising research activity. Similarly, identification of types of families that contribute to delinquent behavior in combination with other factors may prove to be productive. Glueck and Glueck (1970) have combined these two ideas in their latest work with their Social Prediction Scale. They identified three types of delinquents and families from which they come: (1) Core type delinquents who have, among other characteristics, inadequate maternal discipline and no family cohesiveness; (2) Intermediate type delinquents who have some family inadequacies but not as many as the core families; and (3) Failures who came from apparently adequate families. This schema definitely is superficial, especially with regard to recent works on typologies by Quay and his associates (Gerard, Quay and Levinson, 1970) and Warren and her colleagues (Warren, 1969). However, it serves as a beginning in a neglected area of research because it does take directly into account the family's influence on delinquency.

Working with the family to effect changes in their behavior has proven to be extremely difficult. Parents seem to be responding to growing criticism of their child-rearing practices by constantly shifting and bending to please the experts or to conform to their child's expressed wishes. Unfortunately, neither society's experts nor their children knows what is best for the family. If nothing else, until answers are available, parents should at least be encouraged to provide a consistent and clear model of what they believe to be appropriate behavior for the child.

REFERENCES

Andry, R. G.: *Delinquency and Parental Pathology*. London, Methuen, 1960.

Bach, G. R.: Father-fantasies and father-typing in father-separated children. *Child Dev, 17:*63-80, 1946.

Baldwin, A. L., Kalhorn, Joan, and Breese, Fay H.: Patterns of parent behavior. *Psychol Monog, 58* (No. 3): 1945.

Bandura, A.: Relationship of family patterns to child behavior disorders. Stanford University, Progress Report M-1734, National Institute of Mental Health, 1960.

Bandura, A., Ross, Dorthea, and Ross, Sheila: Transmission of aggression through imitation of aggressive models. *J Abnorm Soc Psychol, 63:*575-582, 1961.

————: Imitation of film mediated aggressive models. *J Abnorm Soc Psychol, 66:*3-11, 1963.

Bandura, A., and Walters, R.: *Adolescent Aggression.* New York, Ronald, 1959.

Becker, W. C., Peterson, D. R., Luria, Zella, Shoemaker, D. J., and Hellmer, L. A.: Relations of factors derived from patient-interview ratings to behavior problems of five-year-olds. *Child Dev, 33:*509-535, 1962.

Becker, W. C., Peterson, D. R., Hellmer, L. A., Shoemaker, D. J., and Quay, H. C.: Factors in parental behavior and personality as related to problem behavior in children. *J Consult Psychol, 23:*107-110, 1959.

Bender, Lauretta: Psychopathic behavior disorders in children. In Lindner, R. M., and Selinger, R. V. (Eds.): *Handbook of Correctional Psychology.* New York, Philosophical Library, 1947.

————: Psychopathic personality disorders in childhood and adolescence. *Arch Crim Psychodynam, 4:*412-415, 1961.

Bennett, Ivy: *Delinquent and Neurotic Children.* New York, Basic Books, 1960.

Biller, H. B.: *Father, Child and Sex Role.* Lexington, Mass., Health Lexington Books, 1971.

Brigham, J. C., Rickets, J. L., and Johnson, R. C.: Reported maternal and paternal behaviors of solitary and social delinquents. *J Consult Psychol, 31:*420-422, 1967.

Burt, C.: *The Young Delinquents.* New York, Appleton, 1929.

Carkhuff, R. R.: Principles of social action in training for new careers in human services. *J Counsel Psychol, 18:*147-151, 1971.

Communications Research Machines Books: *Developmental Psychology Today.* Del Mar, Calif., Author, 1971.

Cooper, D.: *The Death of the Family.* New York, Pantheon, 1970.

Dole, A. A., and Nottingham, J.: Beliefs about human nature held by counseling, clinical and rehabilitation students. *J Counsel Psychol, 16:*197-202, 1969.

Douvan, E., and Adelson, J.: *The Adolescent Experience.* New York, Wiley, 1966.

Fox, V.: Psychopathy as viewed by a clinical psychologist. *Arch Crim Psychodynam, 4:*472-479, 1961.

Gerard, R. E., Quay, H. C., and Levinson, R. B.: *Differential Treatment: A Way to Begin.* Washington, D. C., Federal Bureau of Prisons, 1970.

Glueck, S., and Glueck, Eleanor: *Unraveling Juvenile Delinquency.* New York, Commonwealth Fund, 1950.

————: *Toward a Typology of Juvenile Offenders: Implications for Therapy and Prevention.* New York, Grune & Stratton, 1970.

————: *Family Environment Delinquency.* Boston, Houghton, 1962.

Greenacre, Phyllis: Conscience in the psychopath. *Am J Orthopsychiat, 15:* 495-509, 1945.

Harlow, Harry: The heterosexual affectional system in monkeys. *Am Psychol, 17:*1-9, 1962.

Healy, W., and Bronner, A. L.: *Delinquents and Criminals: Their Making and Unmaking.* New York, Macmillan, 1926.

Hertzog, Elizabeth, and Studia, Cecelia E.: Fatherless homes: A review of research. *Children,* Sept-Oct, 1968.

Hirsch, I., and Walder, L.: Training mothers in groups as reinforcement therapists for their own children. *Proceedings of the 77th Annual Convention of the American Psychological Association, Washington, D. C.* 561-562, 1969.

Hoffman, M. L., and Saltzstein, H. D.: Parent discipline and the child's moral development. *J Pers Soc Psychol, 5:*45-57, 1967.

Jenkins, R. L.: The psychopathic or antisocial personality. *J Nerv Ment Dis, 131:*318-334, 1960.

Keniston, K.: *Young Radicals.* New York, Harcourt, Brace & World, 1968.

Lipman, H. S.: Psychopathic reactions in children. *Am J Orthopsychiat, 21:* 227-231, 1951.

Liverant, S.: MMPI differences between parents of disturbed and nondisturbed children. *J Consult Psychol, 23:*256-260, 1959.

Lynn, D. B., and Sawrey, W. L.: The effects of father-absence on Norwegian boys and girls. *J Abnorm Soc Psychol, 59:*258-262, 1959.

McCandless, B. R.: *Children: Behavior and Development,* 2nd ed. New York, Holt, Rinehart & Winston, 1967.

McCord, W., and McCord, J.: *Psychopathy and Delinquency.* New York, Grune & Stratton, 1956.

————: The effects of parental role model on criminality. *J Soc Iss, 14:*66-75, 1958.

McCord, W., McCord, Joan, and Howard, A.: Familial correlates of aggression in nondelinquent male children. *J Abnorm Soc Psychol. 62:*79-93, 1961.

————: Family interaction as antecedent to the direction of male aggressiveness. *J Abnorm Soc Psychol, 66:*239-242, 1963.

Mead, Margaret: A conversation with Margaret Mead: On the anthropological age. In *Readings in Psychology Today,* 2nd ed. Del Mar, Calif., CRM Books, 1972.

Medinnus, G. R.: Delinquents' perceptions of their parents. *J Consult Psychol,* 29:592-593, 1965.

Mennel, R. M.: Origins of the juvenile court: Changing perspectives on the legal rights of juvenile delinquents. *Crime and Delinquency,* 18:68-78, 1972.

Merrill, Maud A.: *Problems of Child Delinquency.* Boston, Houghton Mifflin, 1947.

Miller, W. B.: Lower class culture as a generating milieu of gang delinquency. *J Soc Iss,* 14:5-19, 1958.

Minuchin, S., Montalvo, B., Guerney, B., Rosman, B., and Schumer, F.: *Families of the Slums.* New York, Basic Books, 1967.

Mueller, W. J.: Patterns of behavior and their reciprocal impact in the family and in psychotherapy. *J Counsel Psychol,* 16 (2, Pt. 2): 1969.

Patterson, G. R., Cobb, J. A., and Ray, Roberta S.: A social engineering technology for retraining aggressive boys. Paper presented for Adams, H., and Unikel, L. (Eds.), Georgia Symposium in Experimental Clinical Psychology, Vol. II, Pergamon Press, 1970.

Patterson, G. R., and Gullion, M. Elizabeth: *Living With Children.* Champaign, Illinois, Research Press, 1968.

Peterson, D. R., and Becker, W. C.: Family interaction and delinquency. In Quay, H. C. (Ed.): *Juvenile Delinquency.* New York, D. Van Nostrand, 1965.

Peterson, D. R., Becker, W. C., Hellmer, L. A., Shoemaker, D. J., and Quay, H. C.: Parental attitudes and child adjustment. *Child Dev, 30:* 119-130, 1959.

Pettit, G. A.: *Prisoners of Culture.* New York, Charles Scribner's Sons, 1970.

Post, G. C., Hicks, R. A., and Monfort, M. F.: Day-care program for delinquents: A new treatment approach. *Crime and Delinquency,* 14:353-359, 1968.

Reiner, Bernice S., and Kaufman, I.: *Character Disorders in Parents of Delinquents.* New York, Family Service Assoc. of America, 1959.

Richardson, H., and Roebuck, J. B.: Minnesota Multiphasic Personality Inventory and California Psychological Inventory differences between delinquents and their nondelinquent siblings. *Proceedings of the 73rd Annual Convention of the American Psychological Association,* Washington, D. C., 255-256, 1965.

Riesman, D.: The young are captives of each other. *Psychol Today,* 1969 (Oct.), 28-31, 63-67.

Rubenfeld, S.: *Typological Approaches and Delinquency Control: A Status Report.* Washington, D. C., Department of Health, Education & Welfare, 1967.

Sears, R., Maccoby, E., and Levin, H.: *Patterns of Child Rearing.* Evanston, Ill., Row, Peterson, 1957.

Shaw, C. R., and McKay, H. D.: *Juvenile Delinquency and Urban Areas.* Chicago, University of Chicago Press, 1942.

Siegman, A. W.: Father absence during early childhood and antisocial behavior. *J Abnorm Psychol, 71:*71-74, 1966.

Smith, Judith M., and Smith, D. E. P.: *Child Management.* Ann Arbor, Michigan, Ann Arbor Publishers, 1966.

Stark, R., and McEvoy, J., III.: Middle-class violence. In *Readings in Psychology Today,* 2nd ed. Del Mar, Calif., CRM Books, 1972.

Stollery, P. L.: Families come to the institution: A 5-day experience in rehabilitation. *Fed Probation, 34:*46-53, 1970.

Stolz, Lois M.: *Father Relations of Warborn Children.* Stanford, Calif., Stanford Univ. Press, 1954.

Updegraff, Ruth: Recent approaches to the study of the preschool child. III. Influence of parental attitudes upon child behavior. *J Consult Psychol, 3:*34-36, 1939.

Warren, Marguerite Q.: The case for differential treatment of delinquents. *Ann Am Acad Polit Soc Sci, 381:*47-59, 1969.

Williams, P.: School dropouts. *NEA J, 52:*10-12, 1963.

Witherspoon, A. W.: Foster home placements for juvenile delinquents. *Fed Probation, 30:*48-52, 1966.

Wood, B. S., Wilson, G. G., Jessor, R., and Bogan, R. B.: Trouble-shooting behavior in a correctional institution: Relationship to inmates' definition of their situation. *Am J Orthopsychiat, 36:*795-802, 1966.

Chapter III

FAMILY CRISIS INTERVENTION: A MODEL AND TECHNIQUE OF TRAINING

ROBERTA E. MALOUF AND JAMES F. ALEXANDER

- ■ PHILOSOPHY
- ■ TRAINING
- ■ TECHNIQUES

THIS CHAPTER DESCRIBES the basic elements of a short term family crisis therapy approach which has been developed for treating families of delinquent teenagers (Alexander & Parsons, 1973; Parsons & Alexander, 1973). Three aspects of the program will be highlighted; underlying philosophy, training and supervision models, and the primary techniques utilized. Prior to discussing these issues, however, it must be emphasized that one important aspect of any program development is the utilization of process and outcome research designs to evaluate program impact. However, as the purpose of this chapter is a description of treatment and training approaches, the issue of program evaluation will not be pursued except to emphasize that evaluation is not an alternative but a requisite in any treatment endeavor (Alexander and Parsons, 1973).

PHILOSOPHY

With increasing demands for service from community members, helping agencies (ranging from community mental health centers to school psychologists) are seriously considering the feasibility of short term crisis therapy as a treatment of choice in many instances. For example, in developing the techniques for reducing "soft" delinquency (e.g., runaway, ungovernable, truancy, soft drug use, repeated curfew violations, etc.) in the program described here, several considerations were incorporated. At the most pragmatic level, delinquents and their families typically represent a poorly motivated population with only one third to one half of the cases completing counseling programs. While the often heard explanation for this phenomena (e.g., low motivation, subcultural values antagonistic to counseling, etc.) are probably true, the present program shared the contention of Bergin (1970) and Strupp (1971) that techniques must also be developed to facilitate behavior change with traditionally less desirable clients. To this end the program developed techniques that were understandable, direct, rapid, and (probably most important) produced hope for benefit to *all* family members. Programs giving the message that delinquents should change *for the sake of their parents* or vice versa have, at best, a long uphill fight to face.

This emphasis on the importance of change or benefit for all family members reflects a second major premise, that the understanding and potential change in an individual's behavior is impossible and even meaningless without knowledge of the interpersonal system or systems which influence that individual. This interpersonal systems model emphasizes that an explanation as to why a behavior does or does not occur lies entirely in the kinds of responses it elicits from other members of the system. All behaviors are seen as serving some communicative function within a particular system in that they elicit certain responses from other members of that system and thus maintain established roles and relationships. It follows, then, that if the function of given problem responses is changed and alternate ways of eliciting desired payoffs are generated, the problem behaviors are less likely to reoccur. However, because problem behaviors cannot occur in isolation from the system, it is also important to involve all system members (i.e., the family) in identifying how each member is helping to maintain problem behaviors and generating alternate social maneuvers for each person. The goal of the therapy program becomes the involvement of all family members in their joint responsibility for compromise and change in order to meet and cope with whatever problems arise. This goal stands in contrast to many crisis models in which the goal of therapy interventions is to return family members to some pre-crisis state of equilibrium (Parad & Caplan, 1965). Such a concept, precrisis equilibrium, is not appropriate in families of teenagers who almost by definition are undergoing natural, developmental role changes. Thus in contrast to behavior modification programs with preadolescents, the goal of this program is not to modify specific behaviors (e.g., school attendance) but to train the family in effective problem solving techniques, to adaptively meet the changes inevitably occurring in adolescence. Specific maladaptive behaviors are seen as interpersonal strategies designed to influence the system in certain ways. For example, failing school may represent a way of maintaining separateness in an upwardly mobile middle class family which places great importance on success in school, but in this case would not be the treatment focus per se. Instead attention would be focused on the development of alternative strategies for maintaining separateness which at the same time would not include the maladaptive or "get nowhere" aspects of failure in school.

This example incorporates the third major premise of the program, that of changing strategies, not functions or people. In a short term context, it is unrealistic to think of changing "personalities" or "needs." A wife, for example, who "needs" a more involved husband and uses her daughter's delinquent behavior to force him to assume more paternal responsibility will not easily become an autonomous individual. However, it may be possible to replace the delinquency with more acceptable behaviours that still function to elicit father's attention, and thus continue to meet mother's need. Of course, in this case father and daughter also have "needs," and a similar functional analysis must be made for them. The main point, however, is that therapy is aimed at changing strategies to meet needs, not the needs themselves.

Inextricably bound to the issue of system membership is a rationale for seeing families as opposed to individuals. Regardless of the unit of focus in therapy, the therapist, and often his agency, automatically acquires membership in the individual's social milieu. It is in this fact that defining the family as the unit of therapeutic interest has great appeal. First, it is a more efficient use of time and energy. When working with a client on a one-to-one basis, the therapist has many significant others with which he must deal *in absentia*. In dealing with families, a therapist has a vital, functioning system with which to work. He can watch a family in action, thereby collecting more reliable samples of behavior than if one member described his family, and he can provide a setting in which the family can practice ways of interacting that can be used in natural settings. While individuals can practice new styles too, there is less chance that newly learned responses will generalize and, better yet, be maintained in a system in which other members have not had an opportunity to deliberately select new maneuvers as well.

A second and perhaps even more important advantage of a family rather than an individual focus is the reduced likelihood that a therapist-client-family triangle will emerge. This sort of triangle can easily become a miniature family in which few clear communications are exchanged. Therapists seeing only individuals often find themselves devoting time and energy to produce changes which are only sabotaged by a "malevolent" family. This situation generates blame and fault finding, both of which are incompatible with change. In seeing the client and his significant others, however, the therapist's behavior must be the embodiment of the statement that to help the individual client is to help the entire family. Working with the entire family helps everyone to disengage from fault finding and blaming of any single family member and instead to appreciate the symbiotic nature of the system and the fact that the pathology lies not with the individual but with the interactions among individuals.

TRAINING

Training of new and, in our project, relatively inexperienced therapists followed many of the principles utilized in the treatment program itself. The first experience is in group meetings where trainees are introduced to the fundamentals of the interpersonal systems model, given copies of the training manual, and presented with training videotapes which highlight family and therapist behaviors and roles in terms of the functions they serve within the system. In these early sessions it is emphasized that minute-to-minute communications are of primary importance, and historical data are important only to confirm or reject hypotheses as to consistent family relationships. To emphasize the functional basis of the systems approach, examples are demonstrated where therapist behaviors elicit and maintain family resistance in spite of the best intentions behind their "guidance." This principle is extended to the families themselves, where the functional impact of behavior may be quite different from what was "apparently" intended by the initiator. This point cannot be overemphasized, as trainees typically experience difficulty in avoiding the identification of some family members as the malevolent persecutors, and others as the innocent victims.

The early didactic training phase is soon replaced by live observations via one-way mirrors of therapists seeing families. Whenever possible, trainees first observe one of the project supervisors seeing a family, with another supervisor behind the one-way mirrors providing minute-to-minute translations of the interactions, identifying successful maneuvers, dead ends, and idiosyncratic styles of the therapist. Trainees also observe sessions of other trainees, and after all sessions, group discussions are held to plan alternative strategies, discuss productive and counter-productive therapists maneuvers, role play difficult situations, etc. After four to five weeks in this passive role, trainees begin seeing families, usually with a more experienced therapist at first. As before, direct supervision by supervisors and other trainees continues as do the follow-up group discussions.

In summary, trainees receive much the same experience as do the families they will see: feedback is immediate, modeling and role playing are utilized to change and practice new behaviors, therapists and families are conceptualized as a system in order to eliminate blaming when interactions become unproductive, and the determinants of behaviors are defined in terms of their consequences, not their "intent" or "cause."

TECHNIQUES

LABELING. A major technique involving three facets is that of labeling. In this process the therapist identifies or asks each family member to identify the sequence of events that led to a particular event (in or out of the session). In doing so, the therapist slows the pace of interaction and generates a clearer sequential picture of events, including the part *all* family members played in the sequence (for example, it is often impactful to point out that a particular sequence occurred in the absence of a family member and so that member may play an important part by being absent!). The labeling also sets a stage for subsequent cause-and-effect interpretations which serve to emphasize that more than one family member is necessary for any one behavior sequence to occur or not occur. From this point families are often more willing to see these cause-and-effect chains as modifiable, and to develop alternatives early in the chain.

A second facet of the labeling process is the discovery of inevitable differences in perception and interpretation of events. When it becomes clear that family members perceive the same event in different ways, the therapist can move to the important process of training the family in clear communication and feedback. Such clarity is basic to the process of reciprocal contracting (see below).

The third benefit from labeling is that it allows the therapist to avoid blaming. Family members are seen as "trapped" in a sequence of events that have certain functions, and no one alone is at fault. Family members of course tend to resist this non-blaming maneuver (e.g., "But if he would only. . . ."). However, this noncritical labeling process does set the stage for further negotiation and reciprocal contracting.

RECIPROCAL CONTRACTING. The second and perhaps most important technique in the therapy program is the negotiation of explicit and reciprocal contracts. While the purpose of labeling is to make explicit the patterns of cause-effect relationships that exist within the family system, it is the process of reciprocal contracting that helps the family to jointly develop alternative response patterns. The guiding principle of reciprocal contracting is that the contract must offer some payoff for all involved parties. After each family member is asked for his version of the painful events, the family is asked if the problem they had just described is something they want to change and what *could* (not would) they change. After the range of possible alternatives is discussed, each family member is asked to make a change, *but only in return* for a reciprocal change in another family member (e.g., son attends school if father allows him to use the car on weekends, and vice-versa). It is important also to emphasize that all family members must negotiate contracts (mother-father, father-mother, etc.), not just the obvious troublesome dyads such as mother-child or father-child. Again, this point distinguishes the program from many behavior modification approaches, as the focus is on mutual problem solving (i.e., negotiation for reciprocal contracts) in the family as a whole, not just the elimination of specific target behaviors. In guiding these negotiations, the therapist can insure the new contracts serve to replace the functions formerly served by delinquent behavior. In our prior example of mother's need to keep father involved, she can agree to stop nagging daughter (daughter's request) only in return for father's agreeing to check school attendance (meeting mother's need for involvement). He, in turn, can agree to do so only if allowed to go fishing alone on Saturday, meeting his request to be away from the family at times.

When practicing the art of reciprocal contracting, therapists have several means of determining the likelihood that a contract will be maintained. First the therapist should ask himself the question, "why should I follow through if I were that person? What is the payoff and is it reinforcing for the individual?" Second, the therapist should ask each family member these same questions. Hearing each member describe his payoff tells the therapist how reciprocal the contract is and therefore some idea of how well it will work. For example, if a mother answers, "my reward will be seeing my son be a better person because good boys come home on time," the therapist knows this mother has not yet appreciated the importance of her behavior in the system and the fact that she has needs for herself personally and not just in terms of her son. A reciprocal contract has not been made until each member can describe what he personally will receive if he helps to maintain the contract. An acceptable response from our reluctant mother might be, "when he doesn't break curfew, I don't have to get out of bed in the middle of the night to let him in the house," or "I won't have to listen to him and his dad fight the next morning and then get a headache."

FOCUS ON THE MARRIAGE. Of considerable importance representing more of a point of emphasis than a specific therapy technique is the focus on the parents as a special problem solving unit. As implied in the above discussion, it is crucial that the marital dyad receive special attention apart from the children. The goal in stressing the need for parents to directly struggle and cooperate with each other is two-fold. First, it serves to remove the children from a middleman position in the marriage so that they no longer have responsibility for keeping the married pair together or apart, and second, it reminds parents that parenting is a job that requires both of them to be involved directly with each other in resolving problems. In focusing on parents as a married couple, the therapist steers contract negotiation to include a necessary contract between parents. This does not necessarily mean the parents are asked to no longer disagree with each other but rather to agree or disagree directly with each other rather than through children. For example, a father may want his son to attend church three times a week, while mother thinks this demand is excessive. Nevertheless father expects and demands that mother enforce his rule with son. A goal for therapy would be to remove son from this marital conflict by creating a contract in which father must enforce his own rules with son and agree to disagree with his wife as to the moral value of church meetings for their son, i.e., let them agree or disagree but without son.

Thus, just as the training model emphasized feedback and practice of specific therapy techniques, the therapy model stresses the importance of providing a setting for families in which they all can observe and participate in the process of clarification of ongoing communications and the deliberate selection of alternative responses to each other. It is stressed that the process of labeling and reciprocal contracting are skills that the family can use when problems arise and are not a magic that "good" families have and "bad" families lack. The attention given to the parents serves to bring into focus for the entire family the fact that parents not only have special responsibilities but also a unique relationship and that this relationship, within the context of children, requires direct communications and problem solving.

In summary, then, families of delinquent teenagers are seen as expressing stress (system disintegration in Alexander's [1973] terms) through overt behaviors such as running away and truancy. The family crisis program responds directly to the family's dysfunction through training in concrete, tangible problem solving strategies emphasizing the reciprocal nature of parent-child interactions and the parent or parents as a special problem solving unit.

REFERENCES

Alexander, J. F.: Defensive and supportive communications in normal and deviant families. *J Consult Clin Psychol, 40*:223-231, 1973.

Alexander, J. F., and Parsons, B. V.: Short term behavioral intervention with delinquent families: Impact on process and recidivism. *J Abnorm Psychol, 81*:219-225, 1973.

Bergin, A. E.: The evaluation of therapeutic outcomes. In Bergin, A. E., and Garfield, S. L. (Eds.): *Handbook of Psychotherapy and Behavior Change: An Empirical Analysis.* New York, Wiley, 1971.

Haley, J.: *Changing Families: A Family Therapy Reader.* New York, Grune & Stratton, 1971.

Parad, H. J., and Caplan, G.: A framework for studying families in crisis. In Parad, H. J. (Ed.): *Crisis Intervention: Selected Readings.* New York, Family Service Association of America, 1965.

Parsons, B. V., and Alexander, J. F.: Short term family intervention: A therapy outcome study. *J Consult Clin Psychol,* 1973 (in press).

Strupp, H. H.: *Psychotherapy and the Modification of Abnormal Behavior.* New York, McGraw-Hill, 1971.

Watzlawick, P., Beavin, J. H., and Jackson, D. D.: *Pragmatics of Human Communication.* New York, Norton, 1967.

Chapter IV

THE CHILD OF DIVORCE

Marjorie Kawin Toomim*

■ What Is Lost?
■ The Mourning Process
■ How Can the Child Defend Against Loss?

THE CHILD OF DIVORCING PARENTS must cope with a multitude of losses. While on the surface it appears that he has lost only the easy availability of a parent, in fact he has lost much more. He has lost a basic psycho-social support system. His own dynamic structure has been molded by this system; the fibers of his being have been interwoven with those of his family members in a way which, if not altogether positive for growth, were at least familiar and in some sort of balance. With the dissolution of the structure, the child must now find new support systems.

The process of coping with loss is the same, whether the loss is of a person, a relationship, or a possession; whether the cause of loss is death, divorce, or a marked widening of psycho-social distance (Bowlby, 1961). Losses must be mourned in order to satisfactorily separate from a person or relationship and to allow new persons and relationships to fulfill one's needs.

How the child copes with the loss and the mourning process is crucial to his future development. A certain level of ego-strength, psychic energy, and external support is necessary to

* The author wishes to thank Lillian Freeman and Pamela Kawin for their assistances in the preparation of this paper.

carry the mourning process through to completion. Few children have the capacity for healthy mourning before the age of three and one half or four years (Siggins, 1961). Few children of divorcing parents have the requisite external support at any age.

In divorce, the problem of accepting loss and properly mourning is complicated by the difficulty of discriminating the exact nature of the various losses. Even when the father deserts, his loss is not clear. The child may feel justified in hoping for his return, though, in fact, there is no hope.

Divorce losses are difficult to discriminate. Parents compound the problem by ignoring or denying that such losses exist. Some parents are too absorbed in their own pain to help the child appropriately; some do not recognize the various losses, naively believing that only the person of the father is gone. Parents may even state that the child has not lost his father at all—or claim they will now have a better relationship because they will see more of each other. Where such denial of reality of loss occurs, the parent and the child cannot share mutual thoughts and feelings, or explore alternative ways of meeting needs together. The gap grows wider and losses mount. Parental failure to help in this trying time also alienates the child from himself. The child cannot cope with the overwhelming nature of his feelings. He defends against them. He denies, represses, withdraws, regresses, projects, detaches. He retains in fantasy what is not there in reality and he does not adequately deal with the loss.

Incomplete mourning leaves a reservoir of painful memories and feelings experienced as an undercurrent of depression. A rigid defense system guards against the awareness of ambivalence and pain and is a distorting screen through which subsequent realities are passed, misperceived, and misconstrued. The pain of the loss remains buried, occasionally surfacing when defenses are lowered or "reminders" of the loss transcend the defense barrier. Energy must constantly be expended to hide the pain. Distortion of reality creates difficulties in living; avoidance of stimuli which might bring the pain to the surface leads to a narrowing of life-space. Loss follows loss as the individual finds himself only partially alive, unable to partake of whole areas of existence. Energies bound in denying and avoiding the reality of loss and its associated pain are not available for use in positive growth and development.

Loss hurts; it leaves scars; it diverts one's life-course. Acceptance of loss provides freedom to explore other alternatives in life and to have other experiences. Denial of loss leaves a gaping hole that may only be covered over. There is constant fear of falling into the darkness below. Denial of loss leaves a vacuum in which no substitute relationship can flourish. Needs are left unsatisfied. The feeling of loss pervades one's life. Acceptance of loss and healthy, complete mourning provide a stable base for future growth.

Some of the trauma of divorce can be prevented by advance planning. Divorcing parents prepare themselves by a long period of questioning, expressing feelings, protesting and despairing, exploring alternatives in fantasy or in fact. Much of their mourning process is experienced in the context of the marriage. The child, on the other hand, is not prepared for this major change in his life. Furthermore, he must adjust to sudden loss in a chaotic family setting.

Parents need to respect the ways in which the child copes with divorce. His stress is great, his capacities limited. He does what he can to protect himself from what might be overwhelming stress. The parent may guide his adjustment patterns with tenderness and love, not with criticism and anger. The divorce adjustment takes years, during which time the dynamics need to be worked through repeatedly as the child's emotional strength and conceptual abilities mature. Young children almost universally deny some aspects of their situation. The aware parent can help the child integrate the realities the child brings to awareness as his strength grows. Insistence that the child see the whole reality at once will only bring resistence and move him further into denial and fantasy.

The following sections in "What is lost," "The mourning process," and "How the child defends against loss," describe in detail the complexities of divorce from the child's point of view. They are written to alert parents and counselors to interactions which often occur for children of divorce. With this knowledge and parental self-awareness, the strain of divorce can be minimized. A good divorced family structure may even allow for growth not possible to attain in the failing marriage. They are not intended to deter parents from divorcing—only to help them enter into this new family relationship intelligently and with care. Divorce may be the most important event in your child's life.

WHAT IS LOST?

Loss of Faith and Trust

A tacit contract is entered into by parents upon the birth of a child. The parents, in effect, promise to establish a firm psychosocial base from which the child can grow. In return, he is expected to remain with the parents, to develop and mature. The child in a two-parent family generally expects that the parental unit will continue to be available to him until he no longer needs it. Most parents encourage this belief by assuring the child of their love, concern, and intention to maintain the family structure. Most parents, experiencing a strain in their relationship are especially vocal in such reassurance hoping to allay his fears and "make him feel secure." They do not want him to be unnecessarily upset, just in case they are able to remain together.

For the child, it does not matter how unhappy the parents are together or how reasonable and right that they separate. He only sees that they have been unable to solve their problems in such a way as to maintain *his* security. Even where a parent is cruel or the strain in the relationship so great that divorce would ultimately benefit him, the child has no assurance that his lot will improve. He feels betrayed. He may feel so hurt that he never trusts again. The younger the child, the less he can understand, the more his need for both parents, and the more his need for a stable family unit, the more divorce will leave him feeling betrayed, angry, hurt and untrusting.

The hurt, untrusting child is in the uncomfortable position of needing help from parents who have just betrayed his trust. The likelihood of finding someone outside of the family to help him through this difficult time varies with the age of the child and his level of socialization. Very few children under six years of age have this ability. Beyond six, the willingness to ask for and receive help, the willingness of the parents to allow him to form a closer relationship with another adult or good friend, and the availability of a suitable, supportive individual are crucial factors.

Many children at this point deny their dependency needs and withdraw rather than trust either a parent or a parent-substitute. Or they may remain aware of unfulfilled dependency needs and feel helplessly angry. The child who remains aware of dependency needs and refuses to trust, places himself in the precarious interpersonal situation of feeling unsatisfied and of being unsatisfiable. He has laid the grounds within himself of a double-binding situation that may persist into adulthood where he simultaneously demands and rejects love. As a result, his needs remain unmet and he remains frustrated.

Parents are generally advised (Despert, 1962) not to distress their child unnecessarily by telling him of their difficulties before they separate just in case things can be "patched up." My experience with family crisis is that the child is aware of conflict but does not understand it. Mistrust grows in such an interpersonal setting. Parental honesty builds trust. Parents can be open about the seriousness of their difficulty without burdening the child with unnecessary details, fighting in his presence, or using him in their struggle. Rather, they can *talk about* the fact that they have problems and how they are trying to solve them. The child usually can understand the parents' situation if it is discussed in terms of the child's own difficulties with playmates. Care *must* be taken to understand the extent of his ability to deal with the details of the conflict.

The separation counseling model (see Chapter IX) provides an optimum situation in which the child can be prepared for divorce. Such an approach not only builds trust, but also provides the child with an effective model for conflict resolution. Even the concept that separation may be a constructive step in problem solving may help the child. Knowing when to end a relationship is a sign of strength and success, not of failure.

Maintaining open communication between parent and child helps to build his trust and provides a strong support for him. Only thus can the parents help the child cope with the many changes with which he will be faced as he grows in a divorced family. It is important that parents understand the child's experience of divorce, the logical and moral systems under which he operates at various developmental stages and the ways in which this particular child copes with stress. Without this understanding the parent runs a high risk of being misunderstood and rejected.

Respect for the child's attempts to cope with his difficulties will also increase parental availability and support. The child who feels accepted will be more likely to keep the parent informed of how he perceives the changes in his life and will ask for continued clarification of his thoughts and feelings. As the child develops, he is increasingly capable of conceptualizing and integrating the whole reality of divorce.

Loss of the Child-Mother-Father Relationship

In an intact family, the child has a child-mother relationship, a child-father relationship, and a child-parents relationship. Each parent gives him something; each provides a measure of support, control, nurturance, etc. Together they complement and supplement each other. Even parents in conflict represent a unit. In fact, they represent a very strong unit if, for example, the child has learned to use one as a rescuer when he displeases the other, or if he has learned to gratify his needs by using their divergence to manipulate.

Unless he has assumed a large portion of child-care functions, the father of the infant from 0 to 18 months is more important for his role than for his person. The infant is primarily involved at the interpersonal level with his mother, especially in executing the difficult task of breaking his symbiotic bond with her and establishing his individuality (Mahler, 1971; McDevitt and Settlage, 1971). The father now represents a vital source of support for the mother, permitting her to give the child consistent care so that he may gradually learn to cope with separation according to his daily needs and capacity to tolerate stress. The father also represents a safe person the child can go to as he explores non-mother space. Relating to both father and mother gives him social skills necessary for complex interpersonal relationships. After the 18th month he is able to hold symbolic representations of objects in his mind. Between the 18th and 36th month, he is still involved in the critical separation-individuation processes. Now father loss is important. The child is vulnerable to people coming and going, to marked variations in patterns of living, and to the absence of the father as an individual, not just to his role. The Oedipal experiences of the three to five-year-old are difficult to work through in a disrupted family. The time of the disruption in terms of the child's place in and resolution of Oedipal conflicts is vital. Parental relationships with other potential rivals intensifies the Oedipal crisis.

The child whose parents stay together during the vital period in which basic identification patterns are established will gain ego-strength. Even though parents differ markedly, the child is better able to take from each in an integrated way when they are together. It is also easier to talk about these differences with parents while they are together. Divorced parents seldom are able to talk about each other with good feeling, particularly when value and life-style differences are involved. As parents separate, differences tend to become accentuated and criticized. What the child perceives of his parents is then filtered through this screen of negativity. A parent may be so anxious to pass his value systems on to a child and mitigate the values of the other parent that he pushes too hard. Such an approach leaves the child confused and likely to reject the values of *both* parents.

The older the child, the less difference between parental value systems and the greater their ability to treat each other with respect after divorce, the less serious will be the loss of the parental unit for the child. Maintenance of open communication between the parents minimizes the loss of the parent-unit for the child. As stepparents are added to the child's extended family, such open communication greatly aids his ability to integrate new relationships with their attendant value systems and changes in control and dependency patterns.

Loss of the Predivorce Mother

It is generally the custom for children of divorce to remain in their mother's custody. Therefore, I am going to conceptualize the child's changing relationship with his mother in these terms.

The divorcing mother is in the process of changing her life. She must cope with her own feelings of loss and anxiety. She must find alternative ways of satisfying the needs formerly met by her marriage. She may have to find or change work. She may begin to look for other interpersonal relationships. She probably needs to lower her socioeconomic level, which means she may become less giving of things that cost money while, simultaneously, she is giving less of her time and attention. The child then feels rejected. Conversely, a divorcing mother may change her relationship with her child by turning to him for need gratification. She may begin to spend too much time with him, to use him for her emotional support. Her child then feels smothered.

Many mothers at this time become quite inconsistent. Some quickly try to be "both mother and father," precipitously changing nurturance and control patterns rather than waiting for a new interpersonal balance to evolve. The mother, concerned with her own adjustment, is less available and less sensitive to the child, leaving him with more cause and opportunity to break rules. At the same time that she provides this latitude, the mother may be more punitive or harsh when she does realize that her limits have been violated. Or she may be more harsh because she must deal with control issues when she is overburdened by her own problems. She may then react to her own punitiveness by guilt and overconcern. She may become overpermissive and allow too much freedom because she feels guilty about the divorce or feels this kind of giving will make up for the child's loss. She may be just too overwhelmed by her own adjustment problems to expend her energies in child control. That is something she can "always do later." Perhaps the school or a "Big Brother," or the "father-when-he-comes-over" will do it for her. She may use her energy to get a new husband-father who will assume the child control function for her. Sulla Wolff (1969), discussing children of deceased fathers notes that adjustment was better when their homes were kept intact by mothers who were independent, hard-working, and energetic and who took on the working role with little conflict. She felt that qualities of warmth and affection deemed of primary value for the married mother are less important for the separated mother. Mothers who clung to their children for support, especially their sons, impeded their maturation. Sons of such mothers tended to be tied to the mother and had difficulty establishing a good sexual adjustment.

Personal qualities of mothers seldom change a great deal as a result of divorce. Some mothers feel relieved at the resolution of their marital conflicts and thus are more relaxed with their children. However, if they become heavily involved in dating during this euphoric period their children feel deprived and rejected. Mothers who feel depressed and overburdened by the stress of divorce, though they stay home, are perceived as rejecting by their children. However the mother responds to divorce, the ways in which the child has learned to cope with her are no longer altogether satisfactory. Some change must be effected in order to function well with her again. In addition, the postdivorce child has different needs and so requires new maternal qualities and behaviors. Thus, predivorce reciprocal role relationships are lost, and postdivorce relationships must be established.

Children tend to idealize the predivorce mother; may try to cling to the fantasy that somehow they can get her to change back to her "old self." Feelings of guilt, inadequacy, frustration, and anger arise when they cannot. At times, they believe that the return of predivorce mother will bring the father back. These manipulations of the postdivorce child serve only to create greater stress for the postdivorce mother. She thus becomes even more "different" than she was. The clinging child is further alienated.

A mother who is fairly stable emotionally, has a firm sense of values, and has established predivorce support systems for herself in addition to those provided by her husband and the marriage relationship, is less likely to change much within herself after divorce. She will, as a result, be more accessible to adapt to her child's changing needs.

If the father cannot provide for the family's support, the mother should establish a work pattern and child-care facilities before separation. Thus, her stress is reduced at the time of divorce and the child is given an opportunity to cope with this change within the frame of an intact family. The mother who is unable to cope with the changes in her life comfortably should seek counseling. She thus minimizes the loss of the predivorce child-mother relationship.

Loss of the Predivorce Father

In a divorce in which the father leaves the home, the father-child relationship changes drastically and precipitously. In the ordinary family, the father works regularly, and thus is available to the child in a more limited and structured way than is the mother. After divorce, the structure becomes more rigid and highly limited in time and space. Thoughts and feelings the child may wish to communicate to the father or the sharing of activities must wait until the appointed time. And at that time, both the psychological and the physical space in which father and child meet are often not conducive to the delayed communication or activity. Maintaining a flowing, comfortable, in-depth relationship is ordinarily difficult for many fathers and their children; it is almost impossible under divorce conditions. Time with father is often "time to be close whether you feel like it or not." The closeness, if achieved, must be broken off at the appointed time or "Mommy will be mad" or "because Daddy has other plans for the evening." Many children will not open themselves to closeness under these conditions. Many will not tolerate the pain of repeated separation and loss. It is like reliving the divorce with each contact. Many children are fussy and angry with their mothers after a happy day with father.

On-going reciprocal role relationships between father and child are disrupted in the event of divorce where father leaves the home. The only roles that are traditionally given to the absent father are those of financial supporter, the giver of fun times and extra goodies, and the person who leads the child to much of the outside world through trips, talk of work or business, etc. If the father has held the traditional role of disciplinarian, he cannot do this well at the end of the week or over the phone. Also, he may be reluctant to discipline the child on his visiting day for fear of leaving the child with a bad feeling about him.

In the predivorce family with an active father, his authoritarian role contributes enormously to the ethical-moral value structure of the home. If the father has held the role of rescuer in mother-child struggles, his help will now be rejected by the mother as interference and side-taking unless she actually solicits it. The child may have difficulty accepting the father's help because of mixed feelings and divided loyalties. He may even use such help against the mother or accuse the helpful father of trying to take him from the mother.

The father's role as provider of the "masculine principle" in the child's life is difficult to maintain on a limited contact. Visiting the child or going out to "have fun" cannot replace the feeling that exists when a father actively lives in the home. This feeling is one of almost magical strength and protection against evil or powerful forces. It often transfers from the man to the child, even though by adult standards he might be considered weak and ineffectual. The concept of father as strong protector is further threatened by maternal criticism of the father. Also, the fact that the father does not return or is prevented by the mother from returning home and thus putting the child's world "right" again may be evidence to the child that he does not have the power to help at this important juncture in his life.

Biller's (1971) review of research studies of father-absent sons indicates that the loss of the father as a sex role model has more effect on boys before the age of six than after. Father-absent boys tend to be less aggressive and less interested in sex role stereotyped activities than are boys whose fathers remained in the home. However, the effects of father-absence on sex-role stereotyping may be mitigated by the mother's positive attitude toward the absent father and other males, and by her generally encouraging her boy's masculine behavior. Father-absence does not significantly affect the sex-role stereotyping of girls.

The continued availability of the postdivorce father in part determines how much is lost. However, the child's fantasy relationship with the father may be more significant than his actual presence. For example, an adolescent girl of sixteen had maintained constant contact with her father through wish-fulfilling daydreams and fantasies since his desertion in her third year. The fantasies were reinforced by his monthly support check, one letter and one gift a year, and her mother's constant complaints about him. On the other hand, a twelve-year-old girl whose parents divorced when she was four and a half often refused to respond to her father's daily telephone calls and went with him Sundays only reluctantly at the mother's urging.

Father-absence in divorce is ambiguous. Unless he has deserted totally, he is clearly available to the child at some times. Children believe their fathers could make contact by phone or could come "if they really wanted to" or loved the child enough, etc. The postdivorce father is there-but-not-there. Such a frustrating situation predisposes the child to respond with father-idealization and clinging or with resentful rejection.

Any action that minimizes the ambiguity of the postdivorce father's place in the child's life helps the child. His new roles must be clearly defined. Time commitments must be honored—even if the father sees the child irregularly, he will maintain the child's trust if he is clear about his availability. It is always better if the child and father work out their relationship together without maternal guidance. The mother's role is to accept and support whatever solution they reach.

Many children idealize their divorced fathers as a way of denying their loss (see below). Such idealization, though often hard for the mother to accept, needs to be respected. Both parents can assist the child in expressing and accepting ambivalent feelings. Tolerance for ambivalence is essential to perceiving the father as a whole person, with both positive and negative qualities.

Loss of Environmental Supports

Many divorcing families move from one home to another. Such a move means the child will lose his familiar surroundings. Most children lose a special room in which was found safety, security, and refuge. Older, more socialized children lose friends, school, neighboring adults, perhaps youth organizations and leaders. Environmental supports become more meaningful as familiar parental supports disintegrate. Creating new supports at a time of stress, weakened ability to trust, and negative feelings about oneself is a difficult task. The effect of these losses can be disabling and should not be underestimated. Divorcing families should not move unless it is essential. If it is essential, staying in the same neighborhood reduces the loss.

The Loss of the Predivorce Child

The child, after family dissolution, is not the same as he was before. So pervasive are the changes in his intimate relationships and environmental supports that his feelings and perceptions of himself and others are profoundly affected.

Children are less secure after divorce. They question, with justification, parental ability to maintain a stable environment. They trust less. Dependency and control relationships become difficult.

One of the major disruptions the child of divorce experiences is a discontinuity in identification. Before the divorce, he had been able to assimilate and integrate qualities from both parents with a reasonable degree of freedom. After divorce, the parents are realistically changed. In addition, the child perceives them differently. Generally one is idealized and the other depreciated. Furthermore, if parents criticize each other the child may be afraid to identify with qualities formerly deemed acceptable. With these changes in identification models, the child may now reject formerly acceptable parts of himself which are like a parent he now rejects. He may also experience conflicting feelings about qualities that are now unacceptable to one or the other parent because they are reminders of the divorced partner. Conversely, a child may purposely emulate the qualities of one parent to anger the other, or he may seek to become like the absent parent in order to keep the feeling of closeness. Such major identification shifts cause a changed, usually lowered, self-image.

Most children experience an unrealistic sense of guilt and responsibility about the divorce. This contributes to feelings of failure, inadequacy and lowered self-esteem. Before the age of seven, the child's view of justice is one of retribution. He believes anything bad that happens must be punishment for his wrong-doing. Parental quarrels must be about him; the divorce must be his fault. In addition, the child believes that if his parents loved him, they would reunite, therefore they don't love him. "Perhaps," he thinks, "I am unlovable, what did I do wrong?" The young child's omnipotent fantasies create a fear of his own power as well as an awareness of helplessness. This issue of power becomes central for the child whose parents divorce during his second through fourth year. At this age, a thought is equivalent to action. To be angry with a parent, to wish him gone, and then to find him in fact gone is translated by the child into, "He left because I got angry." The situation is further complicated for the two- to four-year-old in that he often entertains destructive fantasies when frustrated. His inability to conceptualize future time and permanence leaves him the freedom to say "I'm going to chop you up" with little fear. (Stone and Church, 1968.) When, however, loss really occurs, he grows fearful of his anger and magic power. On the other hand, he finds himself powerless to right "his" wrong or to reunite his parents. For example, a thirteen-year-old girl whose parents divorced when she was four announced to her mother one day, "I guess I won't try to get you and Dad together again." This child had devoted nine years of her life to the accomplishment of an impossible task. She saw herself inadequate and a failure. Indeed, so much of her energy was directed to this hopeless project that she had not developed ego-skills necessary for effective functioning in the real world.

In addition to manipulating to reunite his parents, the child may play one against the other or express anger when in fact he feels intolerable fear and sadness. As a result he ends up rejecting parents who care for and love him. He may regress to lower levels of functioning to increase his security. He may feel guilt if his manipulations *are* successful. These manipulations often bring both parental and self-criticism. Thus a negative self-concept is reinforced by those on whom he depends, with whom he identifies, and by himself. The child who feels himself "bad" then clings to parents, seeking reassurance that he is loved and wanted. Such reassurance from parents who are so deeply involved in the child's conflicting feelings and manipulations is seldom meaningful. They often serve only to reinforce his negative self-image.

The stability of the parent-child relationship is threatened by divorce. Before the age of seven, a child thinks in terms of authoritarian morality (Flavell, 1963, Wolff, 1969). Rules are sacrosanct and cannot be changed. What is right for one person must be right for all. Thus, it is not difficult to conceive that if it is right to divorce a parent, why is it not right to divorce a child? If one parent can reject the other for "breaking a rule" or being difficult to live with, why could not the child be rejected for exceeding some limit? He also stays out late, gets angry, likes someone besides mommy or daddy, etc. To tell the child he is not divorceable is difficult, for he has effectively been divorced by the parent who has left him. What assurance does he have that his remaining parent will not also leave? In socioeconomic settings where foster home or boarding school placement is common, such fears may be quite realistic.

A very complex group of feelings is associated with separation from a person on whom one has come to depend. A child must learn to cope with these feelings as he separates from the symbiotic mother-child relationship, from parents and friends as they come and go or from toys as they are lost. In an optimal growth situation short-term separations and minor losses are experienced in such ways that the child learns to deal with the attendant anxiety. Gradually, he learns to depend on his own resources for self-support. He learns to trust that those on whom he depends will be available when needed, even though they are not available all the time. The child from birth through the third year is constantly struggling with the task of separating. Even after this he remains vulnerable to devastation from major losses until he has developed sufficient ego-strength, self-confidence, interpersonal skills and support systems outside of the family to feel that he can survive if the parent is not physically available to help him cope with problems. This level of development seldom occurs before the sixth or seventh year. It may never develop for the child who comes from a strife-ridden home or who has been unable to adjust after overwhelming separations resulting from, for example, major illness, hospitalization or prolonged parental absence. Also, it may never develop if he perceived the birth of a sibling in terms of parental loss. Separation anxiety assails this weakened child at any age when traumatized by the flood of losses which accompany divorce.

Any separation involves simultaneously a complex set of emotions. These include at minimum love, anger, fear, sadness, helplessness, hopelessness and—especially for children—guilt.

Love includes dependency, attachment and need. Without these no loss would be experienced. Perceived abandonment, hurt, frustration of needs and wants satisfied by the lost person or relationship breed *anger. Fear* is experienced in terms of being alone; of further abandonment; of one's own vulnerability; of the possibility that one's own destructive powers may have been responsible for the loss. *Sadness,* the hallmark of loss, is the feeling when something of value has gone and can never be again, the sorrow from impoverishment of the self, the finality of an ending. *Helplessness* is the knowledge that one is not omnipotent; one did not have the power to prevent the loss. Life will continue without the lost person or relationship. *Hopelessness* is the acceptance of the reality and finality of the loss. Even if the lost person returns, it is never the same. The memory and experience of loss alters the relationship. The greatest problem for the postdivorce child is accepting the hopelessness of reinstating the family. *Guilt* usually accompanies loss, especially for the child who still believes he is all-powerful. Guilt is proportional to the perception of his responsibility for the loss, and for his wish that the loss would occur.

How the child copes with this complex set of emotions has a major effect on his subsequent development. The overwhelming force and confusion of these feelings is often too great and he turns them off. He detaches emotionally. Sometimes one of these emotions is more acceptable than the others and this one dominates when any of the others are felt. Thus, his first response to any emotional stimulus becomes anger or tears or fear or sometimes even love. A child can seldom deal with this complex of intense feelings alone. He needs parental support to allow their full expression as well as to gain tolerance for ambivalent feelings.

Parents can provide this support by sharing their separation-related feelings with the child. This does not mean the parent should overwhelm the child with emotion. Rather, the parent can let the child know he also feels sad, sometimes scared, and sometimes glad about the divorce; angry and at the same time loving and needing; helpless and struggling; hopeless about the past and hopeful about a realistic future; guilty and simultaneously justified in separating; aware of everyone's pain.

The loss of inner security and sense of self-worth through divorce is the greatest loss of all. It is also the loss which can most easily be prevented, given parental awareness and skill in helping the child through this critical experience.

Divorcing parents should be particularly careful of the child two to seven years of age. He is most in need of complete parenting and the least able to understand the complexities of divorce. After seven the child is in a better position to adjust. The adolescent has the complex emotional interactions that are inherent to divorce. Also, the adolescent is in the process of separating from his parents. He is the least affected by divorce.

Divorcing parents will best be able to help the child maintain a positive self-image if they accept the special ways he perceives and conceptualizes events in the outside world, his emotional capacities, and his defense patterns. Such accepting parents will be less reactive to divorce related manipulations, emotional outbursts, and defense maneuvers. The accepting parent can control himself and the child better, help him understand, accept himself, and guide him in ways which will build his self-image.

THE MOURNING PROCESS*

The fact that a child's parents divorce is much less important for his future development than how he reacts to the experience. Does he perceive the divorce as a punishment? Does he find the experience overwhelming? Does he compliantly appear accepting while secretly he is angry and too afraid to express anger? Does he rebel openly? Does he manipulate to get his family back together? Does he also expect to be rejected? Does he recognize his losses and mourn them, or does he cover over the pain and leave an empty space inside?

The healthy mourning process involves:

a. Accepting the reality of the loss.
b. Experiencing fully and accepting the complex of feelings which are always associated with loss (love, anger, fear, sadness, helplessness, hopelessness and sometimes guilt).
c. Finishing "unfinished business" associated with the loss: resolving ambivalent feelings, expectations, disappointments, things left unsaid or undone, etc. (Tobin, 1971).
alternative ways to gratify needs are explored.
d. Gradually releasing the lost person or relationship. This may be accomplished in active involvement with the separating person if open contact can be maintained. Where loss is sudden and contact is lost, introjecting the lost one or maintaining a fantasy relationship with him gives the mourner time to master the experience. Ties are then gradually cut while strength develops and
e. Establishing new ways to gratify needs.

---

* For full discussion of the healthy mourning process see Bowlby, 1961; Fenichel, 1945; Jacobsen, 1971; Volkan and Showalter, 1968.

How Can the Child Be Helped to Complete the Mourning Process?

Acceptance is the essence of healthy mourning. Parents can help the child by accepting their own loss and their own loss-associated feelings. The separation process is essentially the same for all members of the family, even though the specific losses differ. The more deeply the parents explore and understand themselves, the better they will understand and support their child. When both parents address their attention to this process, they form a parent-unit for the child. Such a unit mitigates the loss of the child-mother-father unit of the married family.

Parents will help most by focusing on the reality of their child's feelings about his many losses. These are the most immediate in the awareness of everyone concerned. Feelings may be indirectly expressed, but a parent who is in touch with his own emotional experience will be likely to attend to the underlying "real" feeling. Thus, for example, a child who is fussy after a good day with his father is probably sad and defends against this feeling with anger. It does little good to *ask* a young child what he feels, for he has limited ability to put his deep feelings into words. The empathic parent can look at the child's body, his behavior, and his external situation and make some guess about the child's feelings. In the above example a mother might say:

Mother: You looked sad as you came in—before you got angry with me. Did something special happen that made you feel bad?

Child: Oh. . . . No. . . . We went to the zoo and had chocolate ice cream.

Mo: It must be hard for you to have fun with Dad and then have to leave him. I sometimes feel sad after we have a nice phone conversation. I wish then we could have stayed together. Then I get angry because we couldn't. I almost wish sometimes we didn't have the good times, because I feel lonelier when they are over.

Ch: Why can't Daddy come in the house with me when he brings me home?

Mo: Oh. I didn't realize that was important to you.

Ch: Well, I asked him to tuck me in bed like he used to, and he said he couldn't come in the house with me.

Mo: I will talk to him about that tomorrow and see what we can do. I can understand that you would like him to tuck you in. It really feels good to have a Daddy do that, doesn't it. If you will accept a substitute, I would like to tuck you in tonight while you tell me about the zoo.

By this focusing on underlying feelings, the child brought to the foreground one of the losses which was important for him, the tuck-in ritual with daddy. He was able to express his anger about the loss of this child-father interaction. He acted out his ambivalence. It was accepted and a resolution offered. We may assume he felt a sense of rational control over his life and accepted a substitute need—satisfier for the evening. He may also have trusted his parents would work together to give him at least a symbol of something important to him. A fight was avoided and support was given at a crucial time. The child accepted his own needs and feelings as well as effective mothering. Had the mother reacted with anger to his anger, he would have felt less trusting of her sensitivity and caring for him. He would have felt guilty, angry, and afraid at a time when he was especially needy and sad. He probably would have gone to bed pouting, brought his mother back to him with numerous demands (water, blankets, another story, etc.). Perhaps he would have had a nightmare and come to her to relieve his fear.

This issue could have been handled by his father directly. As it was, his mother had to accept the responsibility for dealing with the problem. The father had reinforced his own idealized image as all-giving but failed to deal with the whole child. The following type of father-child interaction would have been appropriate:

Child: Will you come in and tuck me in tonight? You haven't done that for such a long time.

Father: I'd really like that but I don't feel comfortable in the house any more.

Ch: But it is still your house. Besides, you told me you were just divorcing mother, that you were not divorcing me. I want you to come in and tuck me in tonight.

Fa: Wait a minute. There are about three things going on here. Let's get them straight. First of all, I heard you say you wanted me to have some time or do something that would feel close for both of us. You thought about my tucking you in as a way of doing that. Second, you brought up the whole issue of the divorce and my place in the house and the family now. Third, you became demanding and angry, and I started to get mad about being forced to do something for you.

Ch: OK. Forget it.

Fa: No, I don't want to forget it. Let's try to work it out. I miss the things we used to do together that just came easily when I was living in the house, like putting you to bed or reading with you or watching TV. I enjoy our Sundays and the zoo was fun, but we don't have much opportunity to just be quiet together. And you and Mommy and I are never together as a family.

Ch: The house isn't much fun without you. Mommy is always tired and busy now. And she has that other guy here all the time. If she marries him, you can't ever come back.

Fa: Oh, did your wanting me to come in the house have something to do with wanting me to come back to live there?

Ch: Well, will you?

Fa: No, I won't come back. Mommy and I have found that we are much better off living apart, I know it hurts you and that both Mommy and I lose a lot in our relationship with you. But I also remember how much we used to fight and how afraid you were that we might hurt each other. We weren't very good for you that way, either.

Ch: I don't remember the fights very much any more, just the good times. Mommy talks about the fights, but I don't like to listen to her when she does that. She tries to take me away from you. She doesn't want me to like you.

Fa: I can't say what Mommy wants or is trying to do. I think Mommy and I had better get together and work out more of our differences. It sounds as though you are being put in the middle between us, and I don't like to see that. I will call Mommy in the morning.

Ch: OK. But what about tonight?

Fa: Well, I will go to the door and see if Mommy would object to my putting you to bed tonight. But, I don't think that will solve the whole problem. Next week let's go to my apartment and have a regular "Sunday at home" instead of doing something special.

Ch: Could I invite a friend to come along?

Fa: Sure. Now I'll go and talk to Mom.

In this interaction, the father was able to set limits on the child. He shared his feelings of loss; he took responsibility for the divorce with his wife, and relieved the child of the pressure of trying to reunite the family. He took an active role in the family interaction and understood the child's need for closeness with him in a less formal arrangement. The request that a friend join them for the "day at home" is indicative of conflicting feelings about such intimacy. It appears that his son holds suppressed resentment toward him. He would do well to arrange to wrestle with this child during his day at home, or find some other activity that will allow for expression of ambivalent feelings.

By interactions such as the one noted above, communication paths are maintained, trust is built, losses for the child are clarified and defined. The defined loss can be accepted, and substitute gratifications found. Hundreds, perhaps thousands of such interactions are required to accomplish the task of complete divorce mourning. It must be done over and over again.

It is important to recognize that divorce losses change as the child develops. For example, parents who remain so estranged that the father is not allowed in the house will create discomfort for the child at all special events throughout his life where families come together (birthdays, graduations, weddings, etc.). He loses his fantasy of family unity at each of these events.

It is to be hoped that effective parent-child interactions will teach the child to cope with each loss successfully as it comes to awareness. In time he will need parental support only when he is so confused that he cannot sort out the issues himself.

All of us defend against loss because it is overwhelming. Parents must respect the child's perception of his own strength and only help him confront reality when he shows readiness to accept help, much as sexual information is gradually given. He will turn away or misperceive what is said to him if he feels he cannot absorb the reality.

The child needs to finish "unfinished business" with his parents and confront his feelings about them in the present. (Perls, 1969; Tobin, 1971.) It must be remembered that there are actually great changes in the parents as well as the child as a result of the divorce. Children need to work through their "unfinished business" with the predivorce parents in the context of how they were then as well as how they are now. The following example illustrates this point:

Ch: Mom—why don't you ever cook any more?

Mo: I do cook—I make dinner and breakfast and fix your school lunches.

Ch: But I remember you used to be cooking every day when I got home from school. You made cookies and cakes and things.

Mo: Oh that was before the divorce. Now I am at work when you come home from school.

Ch: That is how I always think of you—in the kitchen when I came home from school. I liked the good smells and helping you.

Mo: Sounds like you really miss that part of me.

Ch: Yes. Like you aren't my mother now, 'cause my mother was always in the kitchen when I got home from school.

Mo: You sound sad—like you really lost me.

Ch: I am sad—(child hits the sink).

Mo: Are you angry, too?

Ch: Well—it's not your fault and you had to work.

Mo: No, it's not my fault, but you can still be angry that I don't have time to bake now and that you feel like you lost your mother.

Ch: I don't feel right getting mad at you. You do so much now. I mean, you work so hard.

Mo: Are you feeling that I work so hard that you don't get enough mothering now? Like you are deserted now?

Ch: Well, it would be nice if we could have more fun. You are always so tired, now.

Mo: I miss the good times we had, too. I remember that we use to talk a lot when you came home from school. You told me about what you did and I liked baking with you. I have lost touch with that part of you. When I cook dinner now, you are watching TV and I am so rushed to put dinner on the table I don't cook the same things. I remember that you would chop things for me and stir things that took time. Now I use a lot of frozen food. Asking you to set the table is a lot different from asking you to cook with me. No wonder you resent setting the table now and you didn't before.

Ch: I didn't realize the difference either. And I can't talk to you about my stuff anymore. At dinner now you always answer the phone because it might be a date calling. (Ch. looks away and starts to move away.)

Mo: (Moving toward the child.) I feel sad, too. I don't want to lose you in all the changes that have happened since the divorce. Let's sit down now and see how we can get back some of the good things we have had together. Would you sit on my lap for a while?

Ch: Nods ascent and starts to cry.

Too much was brought forth in this interaction to be dealt with at the moment. Sadness, anger, and love were the dominant emotions. The anger was directed both at the mother and at her "dates."

In a therapeutic setting, the child ideally would have hit some mother-symbol (pillow, chair) while the mother held the child so that the complex of feelings, love, anger, hopelessness, etc., could have emerged together. After the feelings had been expressed, the two could more easily find the closeness they once had. Some mothers would be able to cope with such an interaction outside of a therapeutic setting. Mother and child together would mourn the irretrievable loss of the mother-in-the-kitchen-when-I-come-home-from-school ritual, and find another mutually satisfying activity that would allow two-way open communication. She would also, at some time, deal with feelings of resentment toward the mother's suitors, her tiredness and general unavailability. The child's present needs would be assessed. There may be something particularly difficult to discuss at this time which would have been easier to bring up in the earlier "kitchen" setting. Or, if the time between the remembered interaction and the present is very long, perhaps the child needs some way to regress as a defense against a present stress. The conflict between anger engendered by frustrated needs for mothering, and guilt or overconcern about her mother's additional burdens could be explored. No feelings are expressed in the above interaction about either the divorce or the father. Interventions that might have been appropriate include: "If Dad were here, then things would be the same as they were." "Sometimes I wish we had never divorced. Things would be easier then." "Even if Dad were still here, I had planned to go to work at this time." Also, no mention was made of possible changes in the child's situation. For example: "Then we were so far from people, you had no one to play with. Now we live in a neighborhood with lots of children and you play after school." "You seemed frightened then, and hung on to me a lot. Now you seem to be having more fun with friends. Is that right?"

HOW DOES THE CHILD DEFEND AGAINST LOSS?

Dominant in the constellation of defenses of the child who cannot mourn his losses is either premature detachment or internalization of the lost one or some combination of these.

Premature Detachment (Bowlby, 1961; Deutsch, 1937; Heinicke, 1965) is evidenced by passive withdrawal, active rejection of the lost parent, unusually strong attachment to a substitute, loss of emotionality, or sudden denial of need for the lost relationship. Premature detachment involves a gross distortion of reality—either of the loss itself, or of the child's need for the lost one. Detachment almost always involves a splitting off of intense emotions. It is a most deceptive defense, in that parents so easily overlook the child's underlying pain and react to him as if he were not hurt. Communication is thus blocked and the parents—even assuming they are willing and able to help the child—cannot help. What they do say and do is not addressed to the child's pain and thus he finds it irrelevant and frustrating. He concludes—properly—that his parents do not understand him, and so he further detaches himself from what parenting is available. He grows increasingly isolated and lonely.

The only positive aspect of this defense is that the child saves himself from what he perceives as an overwhelming experience. For him, this is a survival maneuver. Indeed, with it he can encapsulate his pain and deal with it at a later time when his ego is stronger and his support system more secure. Thus, we find adults in therapy working through long-buried thoughts and feelings associated with childhood loss. (Volkan, et al., 1968.)

In rejecting the lost parent, the child may also reject those qualities in himself that are like the parent. Such detachment from himself weakens the child's ego, results in loss of self-esteem and self-awareness, and produces a poor base on which to grow. Some children chose to pattern themselves in any way *but* like the separated parent (develop a negative identification), and thus severely limit growth potential.

Premature detachment from a separated father is likely to result in a too-close relationship to the mother, providing she is available and nurturing. If she is not, the child may detach from her also, continuing to grow virtually parentless.

Parents of children who so defend themselves feel relieved, naively believing that they have easily adjusted. Only some years later do they realize that the child is disturbed and may trace the difficulty back to the time of divorce. The deceptively benign quality of premature detachment is illustrated by the following cases:

Betty was four when her parents obtained an amicable divorce. She was told her father preferred to live away from home because it was better for his work. She saw him every

Sunday. Normally bright and inquisitive, she asked few questions about the change in her family, was easily satisfied by superficial answers, and made no protest about the loss. Apparently she enjoyed the times with her father. He was rather a quiet man who liked to take her to interesting places. She had little difficulty separating from him when he brought her home and she hardly mentioned him between visits. Apparently not concerned about leaving her father when she left the country with her mother at the age of eight, she was quite disturbed about leaving her cat. Her relationship with her mother is close and not lacking in emotionality though anger has not been acceptable in her family. She functions well at school, has few friends. She now suffers from night terrors.

Mrs. I, at forty, has difficulties forming dependency relationships. After her parents divorced when she was seven, she seldom saw her father. Though she remembers their postdivorce relationship clearly, she has almost entirely forgotten their earlier relationship. She is told her predivorce relationship with him was very close. He was a "good" father to her. She has few predivorce memories of him. She clearly remembers an "embarassing lack of feeling" when she realized he left home. In later years she came to resent his abandonment, particularly when she was unhappy with her mother. She dislikes those qualities in herself that resemble his. She has difficulty calling him "Daddy," but easily refers to him as "my father." She abhors men who are like her view of her postdivorce father. She is attracted to men who are like her fantasy of her predivorce father, though she cannot form a lasting relationship with them. After the divorce, when her mother had to go to work, she became quite self-sufficient and absorbed in school work. She became outwardly compliant and inwardly rebellious. Her present rigidly independent stance is a defense against her fears of dependency. She trusts nobody, including herself.

The opposite extreme of premature detachment is *internalization* of the person with the aim of circumventing loss. Internalization may be accomplished by holding a fantasy image of the person or relationship identifying with him (Krupp, 1954) or introjecting all or part of him (Perls, 1969). At the extreme the child may act as if he is the lost person (Deutsch, 1937). The child who internalizes the lost parent accepts the fact of loss but refuses to allow a new relationship to emerge. He maintains control in a fantasy relationship where in reality his control is strictly limited. He continually hopes for something that cannot be. He thus feels frustrated and angry. Underlying his outward appearance of control is his inner awareness of reality and his actual helpless, hopeless position. Internalization of the whole person with both positive and negative qualities is rare. Few children possess tolerance for inconsistency and ambivalence. Therefore, they retain only selected parts that fit a negative or positive image.

Internalization of negative qualities is more likely to occur if the predivorce father was feared. The child then gains power and relieves his own fear. A boy, particularly, may internalize his father's sex role stereotyped behavior in order to resolve conflicts about his own masculinity. If he is not compatible with his mother, he may accentuate his father's negative qualities as a way of punishing her. He may "become" his father to be sent away like his father. Perhaps he takes on his negative qualities in order to force transfer of his custody to the father. Thus he avoids experiencing the guilt involved in actively rejecting his mother.

Internalization of the negative qualities of a parent lead to feelings of insecurity, anxiety, ambivalence, and poor self-image. The child comes to perceive himself as "negative" just as he did the parent internalized. In addition, reactions of others to him are more likely to be negative and thus his self-image is further devalued and his tendency to be fearful, angry, and defensive is increased.

It appears that most children *internalize an idealized positive image* of a separated father, even though he has been cruel or negligent. I recently asked ten adolescent and adult clients from divorced homes: How did maintaining an idealized father-image help you? The replies may be categorized as follows:

1. A denial of the loss. ("I could not accept the fact that we would not be together anymore, so I kept him with me all the time. He was like an imaginary companion." "No one so good could have done such a terrible thing as to leave me, so this way I could pretend it was just temporary and he would be back." "I felt I needed a father, I emphasized the parts of him that I wanted in a father and kept them in my mind that way." "I kept them in my mind as together and happy. That way I didn't have to see them apart. I wanted to have a mother-father unit.")

2. A source of support. ("It really feels good to know that someone always loves you, even if he is 3000 miles away and you only see him once a year." "He was like a Prince Charming who was coming to rescue me." "I kept hope alive by thinking of him as loving and wanting me." "I felt I always had a haven to turn to—a place to go if things got too bad. Of course, I never tested to find out if he would have had me. Now I can see that he would not have wanted me." "Whenever I had a problem I couldn't solve, I would go to my room and have a fantasy in which he came to me and we talked. I did that until I was sixteen—that is the first time I saw him since I was three. Then, after I saw him, it wasn't so easy because he wasn't like my fantasy. I really felt I had lost something." "I didn't like my mother. This way I had at least one good parent.")

3. A boost to self-esteem. ("I must be OK if someone so nice cares about me." "No one wants to come from bad parents." "When my mother criticized me, I could keep from hearing her by thinking about my father and that at least he really cares so I must not be so bad." "Everybody else had a father. I wanted one too. And mine was better than theirs." "It was like he never left me, so I didn't have to feel guilty about their divorce." "I didn't like myself as a person who thinks bad things about people, especially my father.")

4. An identification model. ("I was afraid that if I carried around a bad image of him, I would get to be like that. So

I kept him 'good.' " "I guess I decided what kind of a father I wanted to have, and thought of him that way and then I identified with that image of him." "I don't understand how I got to be so much like him, since I only saw him a few times a year. Well, I am really more like the way I used to imagine him all the time, not the way I see him now." "I didn't like my mother and I didn't want to be like her, so I purposely imitated the good parts of him." "My mother kept telling me I was just like my father. She meant selfish, I didn't want to believe that, so I kept thinking about the good parts of him to be like."

The child who so idealizes the father may considerably distort reality. For example, one girl whose parents divorced when she was four and a half often talked about the "tradition" she and her father had of eating breakfast together every morning. Actually, the father never woke up before noon and seldom talked to her at all. Her mother's attempts to "help the child to see reality" were met with considerable resistance. Already viewing her mother as a rejecting person (the divorcer) and as denying her what she wanted, she became increasingly convinced of her mother's "badness" and her father's "goodness." She then clung even more tenaciously to the relationship with her still-distant father. With so little support for her idealized image in reality, she lived more and more in fantasy.

The child who idealizes his father often finds himself at cross-purposes with his mother. The mother wants to let the father go; the child wants to keep him. She is uncomfortable with the father's qualities; he accentuates them. The child may become unacceptable to the mother both as a mate-symbol and realistically as a difficult child. The child may define as "good" qualities which are questionable. For example, the child may idealize a father's spend-thrift qualities and strain the mother's limited resources and also clash with her value system.

The most positive aspect of introjection of the idealized image of the lost parent is that the child takes control of satisfying his own support needs when his parents deny him such support. He refuses to be a helpless victim. Furthermore, he surrounds himself with a warm, loving, caring fantasy. He protects himself until he feels strong enough to accept the more harsh reality.

Problems with this defense arise primarily when the ideal and the real father obviously differ considerably. Contrast, for example, the case of the girl who maintained a fantasy relationship for thirteen years with a father who deserted her when she was three. She had full control of the fantasy relationship and was only frustrated when her mother faced her with "reality." She had the equivalent to a fantasy playmate or a relationship with Santa Claus. At the other extreme is the case of a girl who saw her father as all-loving and caring and then waited each week for his inconsistent Sunday visit. She often felt betrayed, frustrated, angry, sad, and frightened. She had to repress these feelings in order to maintain her fantasy. The negative feelings were instead turned against her mother, who expressed her resentment at the father's lack of concern.

The child's idealization of the father is the defense most disturbing to the mother. This is particularly true if her own ambivalent feelings are resolved by focusing on her husband's negative qualities (Toomim, 1972).

We may assume that the child himself, while holding onto and becoming like the father, is aware that father was unacceptable. To be like father may threaten his security with his mother. This is particularly true for the child who is told he is "just like his father."

It is difficult for a young child to conceive that parents who are different from each other and who reject each other can both be "good." Therefore, if the father is perceived "good" the mother is likely to be cast in the "not good" position. Parental attempts to manipulate the child's loyalty, change custody, get more or give less money, and to communicate with each other through the child, serve to increase his tendency to perceive one good and the other bad. The roles the divorced parents play also support a dichotomized view. The visiting father takes the child places, goes out for dinner with him, makes up for less time by more gifts and generally sees him only when he wants to and in a relatively good mood. Only the "best" of the visiting father is visible. The mother, on the other hand, increases her role as disciplinarian and has less money to spend than she had when the family was intact. She interacts with the child even when she is tired from working or upset from relationships with other men. She may be seen as rejecting when she pursues her own interests. She is often burdened by her role as single-parent. In addition, she is usually perceived as rejecting or inadequate. The child believes she could have kept Daddy home "If she were better" or "If she wanted to."

Paradoxically, the mother is also a safer person to see as bad, even though rejecting her threatens the child's basic security. The father cannot be taken for granted. He is obviously able to leave and his life is complete in many ways without the child. The child must actively maintain the relationship with him. The child-mother relationship on the other hand is more stable. She has chosen to keep the child, may even have fought for him. Whether she is actually a "good" or a "bad" mother she is a consistent external support who, by her role, gives him many opportunities to channel his confused feelings and gain a sense of mastery over his pain by struggling with her. He wants his idealized father but she is there. He wants his needs met by him; he accepts need-gratification from her. Father abandons him weekly; Mother stays—and her presence keeps Father away and thus frustrates the child. It is difficult to express anger to a now giving father; easy to be angry with a controlling mother. However he expresses his distress—through anger, withdrawal, projection, etc.—the person who will be most involved in coping with the distress behavior will be the mother. Her natural reaction to the child's distress may be critical and thus unsupportive. In her own stress, she may not be aware of his deeper needs for security, understanding of his confused feelings, and relief from pain. His distress is generally frustrating to her. Her natural reaction then is likely to further alienate him from her at a time when he needs her most. He is now very likely to react by clinging to her with fear, and anger while she reassures him. Still full of hurt and righteous indignation, his ambivalent feelings for her grow and his security is threatened by this interaction.

How Can the Parent Deal With the Child's Defense Behavior?

How the parent deals with the child's defense against the pain of loss is crucial. Confronting the defensive behavior directly tends to make the child *more* defensive. Criticizing his behavior or forcing him to "see reality" will strengthen the defense structure and build his conflictful and negative self-concept. He will turn against his mother and make meaningful communication with her almost impossible. Yet, it is important that the child accept the reality of his situation. Only as he accepts reality will he be able to effectively integrate his experience and his feelings regarding his changing family and self.

The way in which parents help their children cope with the complexities of divorce changes with the child's age. Children too young to express themselves verbally can be approached through play materials. For example, clay can be used to create a variety of family interactions with an unlimited number of characters. Clay also has the advantage of allowing the young child, who resists directly confronting his divorce trauma, to deal with it indirectly in third person terms.

Doll play, "dress-up," and role-playing are also good ways of helping the young child work through his feelings of loss.* Snapshots of predivorce family life may be compiled into a picture story which can be read repeatedly to keep real memories alive and in perspective. Postdivorce pictures from both parent-lines may also be kept to help integrate the changing relationships that occur as he grows—perhaps as parents find other mates.

Finding substitute need-gratification is a highly personal task. The parent can help explore alternatives; only the child can know what alternative will be acceptable. Many parents mistakenly believe a stepparent will replace a natural parent. For the child a stepparent may represent a further loss. He may

---

* For more details on play therapy and techniques see Virginia Axline, Play Therapy and also Dibs, in Search of Self.

perceive the stepparent as a rival for his natural parents' time and attention; the stepparent may seem to be an intruder into his relationship with his own parents; the new values and new interpersonal structure threatens old accepted and cherished ways. New stepchildren further erode existing family systems. The problem of integrating such an extended family is a major one.

There is a delicate balance between respecting the child's need to defend against painful reality and helping him confront reality when he is ready. Both parents must work together and with the child to help him see reality as he becomes capable of coping with it.

Divorce never eliminates a parent. It only changes the family structure. For better or for worse a child never loses a parent totally. He has absorbed—introjected—a part of that parent which will always remain with him whether he keeps a fantasy image of him or a real one.

I have focused attention on the basic issue of loss from the viewpoint of the child of divorce. No mention has been made of the child who stays with his father or of the influence of siblings. Too little has been said of the effect of mental age and social maturity and of the quality of parent-parent and parent-child relationships as vital factors affecting the child's divorce adjustment. Unfortunately I know of no research which explores these variables. My hope is that the concepts expressed in this paper will stimulate studies which point the way to effective counseling for children of divorce.

REFERENCES

Axline, V.: *Dibs, In Search of Self.* New York, Ballantine Books, 1964.

———: *Play Therapy.* New York, Ballantine Books, 1969.

Biller, H.: Father absence and the personality development of the male child. In, *Annual Progress in Child Psychiatry and Child Development.* New York, Brunner, Mazel, 1971.

Bowlby, J.: Process of mourning. *Int J Psychoanal,* 42:317-340, 1961.

———: Grief and mourning in infancy and early childhood. *Psychoanal Study Child,* 15:6052, 1960.

Despert, L.: *Children of Divorce.* New York, Dolphin Books, 1962.

Deutsch, H.: Absence of grief. *Psychoanal Q, 6:*12-22, 1937.

Fenichel, O.: *The Psychoanalytic Theory of Neurosis.* New York, W. W. Norton and Co., 1945.

Flavell, J.: *The Developmental Psychology of Jean Piaget.* New York, Van Nostrand Co., Inc., 1963.

Heinicke, C.: *Brief Separations.* New York, International Universities Press, Inc., 1965.

Jacobson, E.: *Depression.* New York, International Universities Press, Inc., 1971.

Krupp, G.: Identification as a defense against anxiety in coping with loss. *Int J Psychoanal, 46:*303-314, 1965.

McDevitt, J., and Settlage, C.: *Separation-Individuation.* New York, International Universities Press, Inc., 1971.

Mahler, S.: How the child separates from the mother. In, *The Mental Health of the Child.* Rockville, Md., National Institute of Mental Health, 1971.

Perls, F.: *Ego, Hunger and Aggression.* New York, Random House, 1968.

————: *Gestalt Therapy Verbatim.* Ogden, Utah, Real People, 1969.

Siggin, L.: Mourning: A critical review of the literature. *Int J Psychoanal, 17:*14-25, 1963.

Stone, J. L., and Church, J.: *Childhood and Adolescence.* New York, Random House, 1968.

Tobin, S.: Saying goodbye in gestalt therapy. *Psychotherapy, 8:*150-155, 1971.

Toomim, M.: Structured separation with counseling. A therapeutic approach for couples in conflict. *Family Process, 11:*299-310, 1972.

Volkan, V., and Showalter, C.: Known object loss, disturbance in reality testing and "re-grief" work as a method of brief psychotherapy. *Psychiat Q, 42:*358-374, 1968.

Volkan, V.: Normal and pathological grief reactions—a guide for the family physician. *Va Med Mon, 93:*651-656, 1966.

————: Typical findings in pathological grief. *Psychiat Q, 44:*231-250, 1970.

Wolff, S.: *Children Under Stress.* London, Penguin Press, 1969.

Chapter V

FAMILY THERAPY IN THE TREATMENT OF ADOLESCENTS WITH DIVORCED PARENTS

AGNES M. RITCHIE AND ALBERTO C. SERRANO

- INTRODUCTION
- FAMILY FUNCTIONING AND DIVORCE
- THERAPEUTIC STRATEGY
- MIT WITH TWO DIVORCED FAMILIES
- SUMMARY

INTRODUCTION

THIS CHAPTER DEALS WITH THE USE of Multiple Impact Therapy methods with broken families, specifically where parents are divorced and an adolescent patient is presenting emotional or behavioral disorders. The authors participated in the development and description of Multiple Impact Therapy (McGregor, 1964) in Galveston and have used this method and various adaptations of it with many families with children and adolescents presenting different kinds of psychiatric disorder.

In the original development of the use of Multiple Impact Therapy (MIT) as previously reported the method was used almost exclusively with intact families. The experience that the authors describe in this paper represents an adaptation to the treatment of disturbed youth with divorced parents.

The use of MIT requires a team of at least two therapists. The procedures include team-family sessions, individual sessions, and various combinations of team members and family members. These procedures provide a structure and an opportunity for improving communication within the family, and for assessment, clarification, and redefinition of roles of various family members. The team relates to the family and to each other in a way that serves as a model of more open and flexible communication and interaction.

It is central to MIT to recognize and to assess family roles, patterns of communication, and of interaction. The disturbed behavior in the child reflects an arrest in his ego development beyond which the family cannot facilitate growth. The role played by each member in the family is determined by their own psychobiological continuity, along with the ongoing transactions between self, family, and society.

FAMILY FUNCTIONING AND DIVORCE

The authors of Multiple Impact Therapy describe four positions of family functioning, which schematically are called: the aggressive (leadership), the passive-aggressive (criticism), the emotionally unstable (spontaneity), the passive-dependent (passivity-cooperation). In well-adapted families these roles function with a great deal of flexibility and of complementarity. Maladaptive families present members functioning in roles inappropriate to their personality, their stage of development, their sex, or to the expectations of the culture where they live. As every therapist knows, growth and change in a patient in individual therapy influences not only his relationship with other family members, but, as their perception of the patient changes, their attitude and relationship with him tend to change. It is our conviction that a multifaceted approach to the group facilitates modification of each member's role performance and the interaction between them.

There are difficult problems connected with communication and inappropriate role behavior in disturbed intact families; these may be multiplied many times in the situation of divorced parents, whether or not either or both have married again and stepparents are involved. The tensions, the disenchantment, and the bitterness that developed, sometimes over a period of years, and finally led to the divorce, frequently have been aggravated by the divorce procedures. These have contributed toward almost insuperable obstacles against meaningful communication, much less collaboration on the part of the former spouses. The adolescent patients had become confused, were conflicted in their loyalties, had developed considerable skill in manipulating the adults involved, frequently had psychosomatic symptoms, and presented antisocial behavior.

THERAPEUTIC STRATEGY

The initial therapeutic goal aims at shifting the area of discussion with each parent from the hostility against the former spouse to a recognition of his or her own concern and responsibility for the welfare of the offspring. The past, of course, provides a basis for understanding the present, but the focus moves to the "here and now" and to the future.

When this shift in emphasis is accomplished with each parent, effective communication between them becomes more possible and joint sessions can be fruitful. Thus, the second objective, the setting of mutually agreed upon goals, can be approached. In no case has the goal been the reestablishment of the marriage. Rather, the goal has been to find ways to provide some consistency and security for the child or children. As the hostile competition between the parents for the loyalty and affection of the children diminishes, some cooperation can begin. As the parents' attitudes are modified, their behavior toward each other and toward the children is influenced. In individual as well as family sessions the adolescent patient can be helped to become aware of his participation in his parents' unresolved struggle. He is helped to mourn the loss and give up omnipotent fantasies and manipulative maneuvers. The adolescent's known strengths are used as a lever to boost his ego identity as separate and distinct from his parents, who divorced each other, but not him.

As it becomes possible for the parents to compromise and clarify their new roles as divorced parents in relationship to the children, his role as a scapegoat loses the old charm, and he is able to deal with his own internal and external difficulties at a more age-typical level.

In each of two broken families there was intense rivalry between the divorced parents for the love and loyalty of the children. The nominal patients were Pauline, the only child of her parents, and Barbara, the oldest of three in her family.

Description of Pauline and Her Divorced Family

Pauline, age 13, developed headaches and abdominal pains shortly after her parents began to talk about separation. Extensive physical work-ups pointed in the direction of minimal endocrine difficulties for which she was treated with no success. She became increasingly anxious, fearful, and irritable. Several months later she was referred to a psychiatrist. She presented visual hallucinations in addition to the previous symptoms. She had a recurrent vision at that time of an old woman coming at her with a knife and hammer. The hallucinations started about the time of the divorce, and seven months after the separation. She became too disturbed to remain in the home and was referred for hospitalization in a unit with an adolescent program (Burks, 1965). On admission Pauline was very restless and anxious. She acted very defiant in an immature way. She said she was "crazy" and giggled inappropriately. She attributed her behavior to her parents separation and implied that she would hallucinate until they would get together again.

Pauline was the only child of the marriage, but her mother (who was older than the father) had children by a previous marriage, all of whom had married and left home prior to our contact. This mother was a somewhat rigid, self-righteous person, who controlled her husband and daughter by adopting a "martyr" role, rather than by the domineering aggressiveness of Barbara's mother. Pauline's father responded to his wife's implied criticisms of him by suspiciousness and by increasing withdrawal from the home for frequent and extensive hunting trips and "evenings out with the boys," mostly his hunting buddies. The climate of the home was a cold one, but the mother endured the absence and the emotional neglect of her husband until she learned of his interest in "another woman," at which point she demanded that he leave the home and she sued for divorce.

This 13-year-old girl, of dull-normal intelligence, had been a rather poor student, but a well-behaved, conforming child, who was described by her mother as a home-loving, "domestic" little girl. She did, in fact, a considerable amount of the house-cleaning, cooking, sewing, and other household chores, so that she seemed almost to excel her mother in such feminine arts. Her father had little hand in her rearing, and apparently spent more time with her after the separation than he had in her earlier childhood. By his own statement, he had little or no knowledge of the interests and appropriate activities of girls aged 12 and 13, and his visits with her usually included dinner and a movie, much as he might have entertained a "date." This suggestion of a "courtship" relationship may have been another factor, added to the usual insecurity and distress of a child whose parents separate and divorce, that caused Pauline to feel more than the usual amount of guilt about the situation, and to become preoccupied with an urgent wish for the reconciliation of her parents and reestablishment of the marriage.

Description of Barbara and Her Divorced Family

Barbara, age 14, was referred for "rebellious and uncontrollable behavior," which included stealing, lying, cursing, staying out late, and going to undesirable places with undesirable companions. She was the oldest of three children born to her parents, having brothers age 13 and 12.

Her parents had married when both were college students, and the marriage was a forced one in that the mother thought, or at least said, that she was pregnant. This proved not to be the case, but she conceived Barbara shortly after the marriage. The family responsibilities imposed by the birth of Barbara, the nominal patient, and two sons in quick succession, interrupted and changed the educational and vocational goals of both parents.

The mother was a highly narcissistic, upward-striving woman, to whom outward appearances were at least as important as realities. To dress well, to live in a nice home in a "good" neighborhood, and to know and associate with the "best people" were her goals in life. To achieve these things she bullied, manipulated, and overcontrolled her husband and her children. The father was an immature, somewhat dependent person, who was bitterly resentful of his wife and his situation throughout his first marriage. He changed jobs frequently, sought to win his children's affection by sabotaging his wife's disciplinary efforts, and generally functioned more like a rebellious adolescent than a responsible adult and head of his household. Their 13 years of marriage were marked by constant tension, punctuated by frequent quarrels. The children, especially Barbara, had learned to manipulate the adults (parents and grandparents) and played each against the others quite skillfully.

Following the divorce, the two boys apparently become submissive youngsters, appearing intimidated by an aggressive mother, while Barbara, just past puberty, became rebellious and uncontrollable and behaved in a way that might have been consciously designed to embarrass her mother. She seemed almost to step into her father's "emotionally unstable" role in the family.

At the time of referral, the mother was employed and was both worried and embarrassed about her daughter's behavior. She was still possessive and controlling of her children, had recently cut short their week-end visit with their father and his second wife, but was appealing to him for help, both financial and otherwise, in securing psychiatric help for Barbara. The father had married again, a serene, warm, apparently stable woman, who seemed able to provide some "mothering" to her husband, and who showed a much more relaxed, accepting attitude toward Barbara than did the natural mother. In the year of their marriage the father was able to settle down into congenial and lucrative employment.

MIT WITH THE TWO DIVORCED FAMILIES

Both girls were hospitalized and received individual psychotherapy supplemented by medication and the milieu and activity program provided for adolescent patients: occupational and recreational therapy and attendance at special education classes in the hospital school.

The parents came in for therapy and counseling sessions on a roughly bi-weekly schedule. Each parent had opportunities for individual sessions with the psychiatrist and with the caseworker, as well as for joint conferences: spouses and parent-child sessions, with one or both therapists. Full family sessions (both parents and child) were usually with both therapists.

At the time of application for Pauline's admission there was so much overt hostility between the parents that an effort at a joint session with the caseworker was quickly abandoned. Subsequent individual sessions with each parent by the caseworker tended to focus on and support the positive aspects of genuine concern for the child, and the wish to appear as well as to be "good" parents. Each acknowledged some bewilderment as to how to be a "good" parent, which provided an opportunity for an educational approach about the needs of a 13-year-old girl, including the need for security in the affection of both parents. The focus was deliberately shifted from the unhappy past in the hope of helping parents to repress their negative, hostile feelings. Reality demands about getting the child to and from her orthodontal appointments provided the first bridge of constructive communication between the parents, and planning for visiting hours, which did not coincide, as well as the coordination of weekend passes, provided a second. The team-family conference on the date of discharge was a calm and fruitful session.

Individual therapy with Pauline focused primarily on her unrealistic preoccupation and hope of being able to effect a reconciliation and remarriage of her parents. As she became in her own and in her parents' eyes more a person in her own right rather than a bone of contention between them, she was able to make a more realistic assessment of the situation. Intellectual, emotional, and physical limitations were carefully reevaluated and found more in the service of the parents' chronic struggle and grossly exaggerated. She was able to move toward increased socialization, ability, and interest in age-appropriate activities.

Both parents were present when Barbara was brought for hospital admission, but the father had arrived the night before, ostensibly because of his work schedule, but clearly hoping to have a conference with the doctor before his former wife arrived, lest he not have a hearing at all.

The treatment program with Barbara's parents was complicated by the more covert hostility between them, under a facade of politeness. They were able to participate jointly in the initial team-parents' conference, to provide history and other information, to discuss the treatment contract, and learn about the hospital policy and program. Individual sessions with the father focused primarily on the needs of his children for some agreement and consistency between the parents about various aspects of child-rearing, including privileges and limits on the children's behavior, and recognition of Barbara's manipulative maneuvers. About half-way through the period of hospitalization the stepmother became involved in the treatment program, ostensibly because tentative plans for Barbara's future included more frequent and extended visits in her father's home. About this same time the mother became engaged to marry and her fiance also expressed interest in discussing his future role with the children, and became involved in the treatment and planning program. The individual work with the mother was focused primarily on her needs and rights as a person and a woman. The courtship period and the evident affection (or infatuation) of the new man in her life decreased her need to exploit and control her children and to deprive their father of their company and affection. Again the emphasis was on the positive aspects of the present and future, with the hope of minimizing or suppressing the negative aspects of the unhappy past.

The milieu of the hospital program was well designed to set and enforce limits on the rebellious, antisocial aspects of Barbara's behavior, while the concurrent individual psychotherapy helped to bring into awareness the self-defeating nature of such behavior and to foster more constructive and rewarding self-interest.

SUMMARY

We have described the use of MIT techniques in the treatment of emotionally disturbed adolescents with divorced parents in selected cases. Results have been sufficiently encouraging to recommend the treatment of the divorced parents, particularly in those cases where both parents are strongly involved in the rearing and management of the child and carrying on their old battles through the youth.

REFERENCES

McGregor, R., Ritchie, A. M., Serrano, A. C., et al.: *Multiple Impact Therapy with Families.* New York, McGraw-Hill Book Company, Inc., 1964.
Burks, H. L., Serrano, A. C.: The use of family therapy and brief hospitalization. *Dis Nerv System,* Vol. 26, December, 1965.

Chapter VI

PREDICTION OF DELINQUENT BEHAVIOR*

HENRY RAYMAKER JR.

■ EARLY DELINQUENT MANIFESTATIONS
■ NEED FOR PSYCHOLOGICAL EVALUATION
■ JUVENILE DELINQUENTS AND PROJECTIVE TECHNIQUES
■ NEED TO BE SENSITIVE TO ORGANIC FACTORS
■ SELF-CONCEPT AND THE JUVENILE DELINQUENT
■ COMMUNITY RESPONSIBILITY

A T A TIME WHEN CRIME RATES are increasing, especially in of-
fenses by young people, a review of signs of juvenile delinquency or indices of prediction, along with a review of the contribution that a practicing psychologist can make, is appropriate.

The detection of early signs of delinquency is most likely to
occur in the home and school. The loss of interest in school subjects and conflicts with authority figures in the home and school
often precede some acting-out behavior which finally force society to respond and make an official case of juvenile delinquency. It is the sensitivity and motivation of the teachers to make
referrals to guidance centers and professionals and the willingness of parents to seek help when these early signs are detected
that could lead to a reduction and prevention of juvenile delinquency. Also, parents who are sensitive to early manifestations
of delinquent behavior can take corrective action.

---

* Taken from Cull, J. G. and Hardy, R. E. (Eds.): *Climbing Ghetto Walls.*
Springfield, Ill., Charles C Thomas, 1973.

EARLY DELINQUENT MANIFESTATIONS

Some of these early signs are resentment of authority figures in the home and school and overt conflicts, resentment of overprotection, resentment of limits and discipline, loss of interest in school subjects and obvious underachievements, confusion associated with inconsistent discipline, impulsiveness associated with permissiveness, suggestibility associated with peer group antisocial influences, frustration in the child and a need for compensatory behavior, compulsive stealing associated with poverty, involvement with drugs which usually has emotional and social motivations, etc.

There are many ways a child or adolescent may show tendencies toward delinquency. Also, in each case there are different origins, meaning and a matter of degree. The practicing psychologist, counselor, teacher, parent and society are faced with understanding multiple forms of delinquency and multiple causes that require an individual and clinical approach.

NEED FOR PSYCHOLOGICAL EVALUATION

To understand a youth and his behavior and formulate predictions, a psychological evaluation of the intelligence, achievement, personality and feelings of the youth, along with a family and social history, is necessary. This provides the evidence to determine causes and early signs, needs, frustrations, infer predictions, and plan treatment or guidance.

The majority of young people who come to the attention of psychologists and court workers appear to have normal or average intelligence. Determining this dimension of the youth's profile can make our predictions and placement realistic and will maximize success. We do often see in this population underachievement in school subjects. Evidence that the youth is functioning below his native or potential level, such as observing that his achievement scores are often below his I.Q. and grade placement, can identify problems which when corrected may prevent delinquency. Many delinquents are functioning below their ability level, and are behind in their achievement. One great need which exists in our school systems is to reach these children with remedial instruction and the possibility of these resources existing influences our predictive judgment.

In cases where the juvenile delinquent is mentally retarded and this is confirmed by individual intelligence testing, we can often reduce or control delinquency by removing a major source of frustration by placing the child in a special class within the school system for educable mentally retarded children. This reduces the stress and the feelings of rejection that the retarded child shows, which often is the frustration that causes his delinquency or aggression. The success and acceptance that the retarded child feels in a special class may meet the need that will modify the behavior pattern and increase conformity. Consistent discipline, structure, and appropriate school placement appear to be the treatment needs of the delinquent who is mentally retarded and at the appropriate age referral to the vocational rehabilitation agency is needed. The degree that these resources exist in the community is relative to predicting the behavior of the child.

JUVENILE DELINQUENTS AND
PROJECTIVE TECHNIQUES

In the evaluation of the adolescent a sensitive instrument, which provides the psychologist with a sampling of the youth's feelings, attitudes and types of identifications, is the Thematic Apperception Test, or projective technique. The themes and stories which the youth creates on the picture cards in this technique provide meaningful insights into the youth's underlying identifications, feelings and often reveal long felt frustrated needs. Documentation in these areas may identify signs of the degree of the delinquency trend and needs in the youth's personality that are relevant to prediction and management. Experience shows that projecting hostility and aggression is often one of the most frequent themes that a delinquent develops in the stories he creates on this test.

A second frequent theme is the fact that many youths identify with human figures who are depressed and are moody, introspective, or resentful in areas of authority, restrictions, rejections, etc. A third frequent theme is the fact that many youths also project a need to be successful and identify with human figures who are striving for success and recognition. An observation that we frequently see in average or bright adolescents who are in custody because of their delinquency is an admission of faults and acts of delinquency and projecting desires to be a better and more successful person. They try to give the impression that they have learned their lesson and are going to try to do better.

Sometimes these adolescents show abilities at manipulating. Often, however, their comments suggest an awareness of guilt and a need for help. These are content areas where a majority of juvenile delinquents usually project feelings and attitudes on the Thematic Apperception Test and can be one of the most helpful clinical techniques that the practicing psychologist can utilize.

NEED TO BE SENSITIVE TO ORGANIC FACTORS

In the battery of tests used by the psychologist are also measurements that can identify organic brain dysfunctioning. In a small minority of these cases some subtle organic deficit may be partially responsible for aggressive or antisocial behavior. In addition to the tests of intelligence and personality, a sensitive instrument in detecting organicity is the Bender Gestalt test where the child has to copy on paper a series of geometric designs. It is important to rule out organic damage or factors and when identified referral to medical consultation and appropriate treatment and planning may control the aggressive behavior of the child. These awarenesses also help the teacher, counselor and parent to better understand and relate to the child. These determinations are relevant to predictive judgments on the course of the child's behavior and adjustment.

SELF-CONCEPT AND THE JUVENILE DELINQUENT

In predicting the behavior of the juvenile delinquent or estimating response to treatment it is useful for the practicing psychologist to determine the self-concept of the youth. The delinquent usually shows inadequate self-confidence or sees himself in negative ways and overcompensates for these feelings by being openly aggressive and hostile. The delinquent who maintains a negative self-image may continue to behave accordingly as a way of expressing hostility. It is the analyses of the origin of these perceptions and emotions that often are helpful in achieving self-awareness and insight and permit the delinquent, psychologist, counselor, and others to take steps to resolve and modify these behavior patterns.

The practicing psychologist may be able to infer the self-concept of the youth from the youth's identifications and projections on the Thematic Apperception Test. As a supplement to this, a practical approach to determining these self-perceptions is to ask the youth to write a letter about himself indicating how he sees himself, how he sees his problems and how he feels. Also, it is useful to have the youth complete a sentence completion test as many self-concept projections are revealed by this approach.

Therefore, the practicing psychologist's approach to the problem of juvenile delinquency and the study of prognostic signs is a responsibility to evaluate the intelligence and personality of the child or adolescent, determine his needs, attitudes, feelings, self-concept, review the social history, make recommendations, and be available as a treatment consultant.

It is in the focusing of the recommendations that a sensitivity to the indices of prediction is important as we strive to reduce delinquent behavior patterns. That is, the psychologist needs to make recommendations that may reduce the frustration in the child's life or meet the particular needs in each unique case that will remove the causes of delinquency. It is necessary that the community plan resources that can follow through on these recommendations. They usually include a progressive juvenile court, child guidance clinics, special education classes and consultation with the school system, social agencies such as rehabilitation services, and professional personnel working together in effective communication and coordination.

A psychological evaluation in isolation of the child's environment and continuing influences and resources is an academic exercise. When needs are documented and resources in the community are lacking, then it is the success which we achieve in getting community and social action to develop these resources that will make each community a low predictive or a high predictive environment for success in reducing juvenile delinquency.

In order to formulate or identify signs or indicators which may be used to infer predictions the clinical case method does reveal a pattern or similarities which suggest areas that are relevant in the etiology, treatment, prognoses and prevention of juvenile delinquency. The inferences from this practical experience can offer some indices of prediction. Also, possible warning or early signs in the general preschool and elementary school age population can assist us when parents, teachers and society respond and try correcting problems or meeting frustrated needs before delinquent behavior is manifested or comes to the attention of the court.

COMMUNITY RESPONSIBILITY

It is through a mental hygiene and public health principle of prevention that the magnitude of the juvenile delinquency problem in society must eventually be approached. Juvenile court judges are becoming more aware of the significance of meeting needs, arranging for individual and family counseling and treating the emotional dynamics of delinquency. In this corrective and rehabilitative process the involvement of family, school and supportive service agencies working together can increase the prospect of success as more people see the need for treating causes, frustrations and emotions in contrast to simple removal or isolation of the delinquent from society. It is in the area of social change such as the removal of double standards or the inconsistencies in society that additional progress can be made, as often many causes and signs of delinquency are related to poor examples of adults.

A community which is a dynamic society and progressive can cope with problems of juveniles and create a more favorable environment. The worker in this field needs to be involved in social change as behavior is a function of internal and external motivation and influences.

In summary, juvenile delinquency can be reduced by a community sensitive to early signs and indices of prediction of delinquency and can take corrective action. Also, the child who becomes involved in juvenile court action can be evaluated and helped to become a more satisfied and productive person as the sources of his frustrations are removed by planning and counseling.

A forthright approach is for the community to recognize its problems and try to communicate and offer services for this important group of young people, correct its own shortcomings by removing inconsistencies or double standards, provide healthy identifications for youth and provide adequate education, recreation and guidance facilities.

Chapter VII

COUNSELING THE PARENT OF THE CHRONIC DELINQUENT*

JEROME ROSENBERG

- CHRONIC DELINQUENCY AND THE ROLE OF THE PARENT
- I. SUPPORT INTERVENTION
- II. CHANGE INTERVENTION
- III. COMBINATION SUPPORT-CHANGE INTERVENTION

WITH THE GROWTH of our understanding of the factors involved in the development and maintenance of behavioral difficulties, we have come to realize that effective attempts at modification of behavior must now go well beyond the individual who has the specific problems. In this sense we no longer speak about simply a patient or a client, but rather we must place this individual in the context of the environment in which he lives, his family, his society, etc. Consequently, in looking at the problems of behavior of children we have begun to realize that unless we are willing to make the effort to work with the parents and with the school, if the child is of school age, then any effective treatment will be markedly limited. So it is in working in the area of delinquency. Unless we are willing to look into the conditions that produce delinquency, the environment of the home and the interrelationship between the individual delinquent and his parents and all other variables of associations

---

* Taken from Cull, J. G. and Hardy, R. E. (Eds) : *Climbing Ghetto Walls.* Springfield, Ill., Charles C Thomas, 1973.

that include this child, we will expend great efforts in treatment with very little positive long-term results.

The model for this chapter will be aimed at the following specifics. First, we will look at the concept of chronic delinquency and procedures for assessing the role of the parents in the particular family situation. Second, we will look at the concept of support intervention in which the major focus of the person involved in working with the family will be to support the parents in adjusting to the particular problems presented by their child. Third, we'll look at a model of change intervention where the focus will be to work with the parents to significantly alter their relationship with their child. Fourth, a dual model in which the focus will be to support the parents in terms of their role in the family situation but also to teach them some basic skills in which they can now work more effectively with their child. Finally, we will summarize and tie the various materials covered together.

CHRONIC DELINQUENCY AND THE ROLE OF THE PARENT

It is obvious by the specific title of this chapter that we are talking about a situation in which the individual delinquent child is a repeat offender to the extent that we can apply the word chronic to describe his overall behavior. Essentially we are saying that whatever attempts have been made to control this behavior in the past have proven to be unsuccessful, and he remains in constant trouble with various authorities in society. In speaking about chronic delinquency we are talking then not about attempts at prevention of delinquent problems, for obviously the problems have been well developed, but we are talking very specifically about an intervention model; an attempt to move into an already existing set of problems and remediate those problems to whatever degree is possible. Our focus here in attempting to remediate is to first understand what is the role between the delinquent in the family, male or female, and the parents. Now here, obviously, the initial assessments to be made by the intervener is the determination of what constitutes the family. This would include whether both parents are living at home, how many siblings, relatives, grandparents, etc., are living within the family constellation. This is important since all of them play an integral part in the maintenance, development, and the hopeful remediation of the problem of the delinquent.

Once we have made this very basic determination, we must then begin to look into the interrelationships between the various members of the family and the delinquent. In doing this, what is required is more than simple interviews with the parents and the delinquent in one's office. What is required here is home visitation, in which the individual who will be working with this child and the parents, will visit the home and spend time in the home observing the interrelationships of behavior within the household. It is very important to carry out this work in the home environment so that there is a chance for concrete changes in behavior under the conditions that those behaviors are most likely to occur. It is clear that any attempts at therapy within a therapist's office is done under the very artificial situations created by an office, in which the behaviors that occur are often very different from those that are creating the problems in the home environment. Therefore, while information must be gained from the parents in terms of their perception of the home situation and from all other people who have data to bring to the therapist in terms of the home environment, it is critical that direct observations be made, and that they be made more than once so as to guarantee that there is some degree of reliability of the data that has been collected, and some degree of validity concerning what was observed, and that it was not simply created for the benefit of the therapist.

At this point it is important to mention the need for collecting and keeping accurate records concerning specifics of the case on which you are working. Very often records that are tuned to the observations and data collected, particularly on home visitation, can be invaluable in coming up with an effective intervention program that will begin to produce positive changes in the environment in which one is working. In collecting data and in attempting to assess the specifics of the problems, a number of very basic questions must be asked; for how they are answered very often will determine what is the best course of intervention for this particular situation.

The first basic question is concerned with the behaviors that are occurring within this family situation, since the primary concern here is counseling the parents of the delinquent. What then are the behaviors of the parents at this point, in terms of how they relate to and work with their children? Particularly, what are the behavioral patterns of the relationships between the delinquent and his parents or whoever is there within the role of the parents? This means attempting to define as clearly as possible what the interactions are in terms of what does the young child do, how do the parents react to it, how does the child react to them and how does this continuous interaction lead to whatever difficulty may be faced by both parents and the child, at this moment.

In attempting to define the problem, it is also very important to understand just how often the difficulties are occurring. As we look at the particulars of the home situation, we may find that very often it is not so much the specific behavioral interactions that are the problem, but rather the frequency with which they occur. The goal of treatment that is eventually determined for this situation may be not eliminating a behavioral interaction, but reducing how often that behavioral interaction occurs. It is also possible that if it is a good behavior interaction, then treatment will be to increase the frequency with which it occurs.

So we are looking first to define behavioral interactions between the parents and the delinquent, and second, to determine just how often these interactions are occurring. From this, the determination of increasing, maintaining, or reducing these interactions can be made by the person who will be intervening to produce some behavioral changes.

Having defined the behavioral interactions and having gained information on the frequency of occurrences, it is very important to understand what the conditions are in the home environment under which these specific behavioral interactions are occurring. Are there specific situations that lead to specific behaviors or do we find that the interactions between the parent and the child are so pervasive as to defy easy analysis in terms of times of day or what antecedent events may have occurred to lead to this situation? This information is particularly important in terms of helping to focus in on what kind of variables may be occurring; if we could control those variables we might in fact be able to control much of the behavior problem.

To review, the basic questions in defining the behavioral interrelationships between the delinquent and his parents are: (1) What are the behaviors that define the relationships and interactions between parent and child (both good and bad)? (2) What are the frequencies with which their behavior occur? and (3) What are the conditions under which their behavior occur? Now we can go one step further. What kind of variables seem to be maintaining the problem behaviors? Here again we are looking for information that may be available to us and narrow it down so that it leads to some specific prescriptions of treatment. In asking what maintains the behavior, we are concerned with situations in which the parent's reaction to the child serve as a major reinforcer for the child to engage in that same behavior again.

This is particularly true if the child is trying to "bait" the parents; if the parents react as the child expects and desires, one could predict from our knowledge of behavior, that the chances for the child baiting the parents in the future is very high. Therefore, it is the parent's behavior that is maintaining the problem interaction. Again, valuable information to help us define and set up our intervention procedure has been obtained. We can now add the fourth question to our list: (4) What is maintaining the problem behavior?

Having obtained specific data from our observations of the parent and the delinquent's interactions, it is now important to sit down and begin pulling together the picture that has been developed in terms of the environment of the child, particularly the home situation. It is often easy to find obvious problem areas in a home situation, for we know a great deal about the kind of environments that tend to produce delinquency and I think as you look through the various other chapters in this book you will find a wealth of information in understanding many, many variables contributing to delinquent behaviors.

For the purpose of intervening in the home situations and in working with the parents in attempting to develop a means by which they are able not only to find more pleasure in their own lives, but to be more effective in working with the problems created by the chronic delinquent in the family, it is important to focus in on those things that seem to have the highest visibility in terms of problem areas. One factor which is very important in attempting to intervene in any situation is getting some success early in your program. This can go a long way toward winning both the support, the enthusiasm, and the commitment of the parent; not only to continuing the program, but to working more actively to see it succeed. The parents have come to you for help. In that sense at least part of the battle has been won. That is, they recognize the need and they have determined that you are somebody, by virtue of your training who can fill the need.

Now we must also recognize that many parents have come to you by way of the courts, so they may be markedly reluctant to offer any help in whatever you might want to do. This again is part of the data that your observations and interviews with the parents and your home visitation will have given you. And this is part of the assessment you must make to determine what role you will take in working with the parents. You must determine what difficulties you will have in attempting to get the parents to work with you and the best strategy that you could use to go about developing the necessary kind of conditions to allow your intervention to begin. You must then tie this all together, particularly the definition of the problem, the frequency of the occurrence of the problem, the conditions under which it occurs and what you have determined seems to be maintaining this behavior, so that you can be comfortable in your position as the help agent. Now you are in a position to make some determination as to what your strategy will be.

This leads us to the next three areas.

1. SUPPORT INTERVENTION—First, the parent is functioning at

a very high level of efficiency and it would appear that all their best efforts; efforts that you would support, are not working. Consequently, the parents do not need to be taught new techniques but rather need to be given the necessary support to allow them to continue to do the work they are doing, allow them to find something within this situation that is positive for them to work with and to help them through the continuous crises situation that are defined by the chronicity of the delinquency problem.

2. Change Intervention—The second alternative is that your assessment of the family situation has determined that the parents are basically ineffective in what they are doing and they need to be taught specific techniques that will allow them to effectively work with their child. Here your role will be partially an educator and partially a therapist because your ultimate focus is to get them to be more effective at how they work with their child. The amount of time available for you to work with the parents or the child is markedly limited, but if you are successful with the parents they have their whole future to work with this youth.

3. Support-Change Combination—The third option left open to you; based upon your initial assessment of the family situation, is that the parent not only needs to have basic techniques taught to them but they have tried very hard and need a great deal of support to continue the efforts and support for them to make the attempt to learn a new approach and to carry it out. This can be seen as a combination program of both support for the parent and teaching them to use new techniques to handle the old chronic problems that they have been having to face.

I. SUPPORT INTERVENTION

In situations where the delinquency problem is a chronic one, it would seem obvious that the amount of energy, the investment of time, and the amount of stress that the parents have been through will have been both long in duration and high in frequency. Consequently, it is very likely that the parents of the chronic delinquent will be very close to that point in which they will not only be markedly inefficient in how well they work with the delinquent, but at the point in which giving up (condemning themselves as losers and as poor parents) is very close if not already reached. Therefore, probably in all programs of intervention and working with the parent of the chronic delinquent, it will be necessary for some supportive role to be played by the therapist.

Total intervention on the part of the therapist is best handled by a straight, total supporter role, and would be based upon an assessment of the situation in which the efforts of the parents have been good efforts. The programs that they have worked with have under the circumstances, been good programs. The parents have not lacked for an involvement with the child, but as is true in so many of our delinquency cases today, delinquency is unexpected, based on looking into the home in which there tends to be many, many positive factors that simply would not be predictive of delinquency. Therefore, this parent needs a great deal of supportive counseling on the part of the therapist; part hand-holding and part recognition that they deserve to be reinforced for their continuous efforts to this point.

It is also important to help them understand and assess honestly their role in the problem so they do not feel a stronger sense of guilt than may be appropriate for the situation. It is important that they understand that all their efforts, however inefficient and however difficult they may have seemed in the past, probably have maintained the situation so that it has not gotten any worse than it is. They should also understand that their commitment as parents is being met at the highest level and there are many circumstances in which the love, faith, and the help of the parent simply have proven to be not enough to control certain behaviors that develop under influences that the parents simply do not have enough control over. By proving these things to the parents it will help them continue to see themselves in a positive role in working with their child.

Also, the therapist's supportive role will be in terms of the kind of things the parents want to continue doing. They should feel free to talk with the therapist concerning changes in their attitude that they think might be affective in working with their child. And again, the likelihood that the parents will find themselves continually involved with various authorities, police, courts and probation officers, they will need somebody not only to support them in their continuous on-going crisis situation, in the chronic aspects of never knowing what will happen next, and in the constant pressure of meeting demands placed on them by the courts and others; the support of somebody who can convey to them necessary information to understand the judicial system, the court system, and the police role will also be needed.

I think that in working with many parents you find ignorance of what is happening contributes to much of the real stress. When the parents are well-informed of what is happening however, they may have no control over the situation, but they are much more capable of coping with their own needs as well as those of the chronic delinquent.

The frequency of contacts of the supportive program should be determined by the initial assessment. If the parents are at a critical point in their involvement and need to be seen very frequently, then I think visitation should be done as often as possible. Again, crisis intervention becomes a very critical kind of thing and support is being available—whether it is a call or a visit in the middle of the night. Sometimes, just being available is one of the strongest supports a parent can have, because they always know that there is somebody who cares, somebody who is willing to listen and somebody who is willing to put out an extra effort to help them.

As determined by the initial assessment, additional supportive measures will be determined by the degree of the problem, by how long it has been going on, by what immediate factors are present in the situation and what long term factors need to be considered. Probably one visit a week on the average would be sufficient for most situations. Many visits could be every two weeks, some once a month, and some even longer than that. Other cases may need to be seen two, three times a week or some even more.

It is clear that with the development of crisis intervention centers throughout the country a twenty-four hour a day phone line can be invaluable in handling immediate crisis situations that come up at times in which agencies are usually unavailable. If there is a crisis intervention program available in your community the parents should be made aware of it. If no such program is available, then you as the therapist probably should be available when necessary on twenty-four hour call. What is important is that the parents in need have somebody to support them, to be there to back them up when problems occur and to know that they can count on you. And in that sense, just being there can mean a great deal of difference in how well they are able to handle not only the day-to-day problems that they must face, but those constant crisis situations that all too often will be sprinkled in with the continuous chronic problems created by the delinquent situation.

It is important to recognize that while some distinction is being made between kinds of intervention, it is highly possible for one particular intervention technique to move into another, as conditions in the situation change and as you are able to gain more information and knowledge of the interrelationship between the parents and the delinquent youth. It is important to recognize that how you do the specific interventions of the supportive program are determined by your viewpoint on therapy, but even more critically, by the data you collected in assessing what the problem was. Therefore, to give you a rote supportive model is to do an injustice to the data you collect and the need for you to be responsive to the problem as observed and defined by you during the course of your early interviews and home visitation.

Again, recognizing the need to be responsive to your data and to the changes in your observation, it is highly likely that movement from a supportive model to a change intervention model can occur at any time; depending upon the specific behaviors of the chronic delinquent in the family and the changing environmental conditions that occur because of the delinquent's behavior. Consequently, let us now look at the change intervention model.

II. CHANGE INTERVENTION

With the major focus of the intervention model being to change the manner in which the parents themselves behave as it relates to the delinquent in the family, there are two methods that can be used to bring about this change. The choice is dependent in part upon the kind of relationship that has been established between you as a therapist and the parents over the period of time you have been working with them.

The first method would be based upon a well-developed mutual trust so that you can clearly show the parents what they are doing and that at the moment is not being effective in helping the child. You can give them a strong awareness of their current behavior and begin developing in them an appreciation for alternative patterns of behavior that they might use as it relates to specific examples that you are able to demonstrate. Here it is very critical that you offer the parent something that they can point to, acknowledge and begin to use as a means of measureing the degree of change they are able to accomplish.

The second particular model is based upon a situation in which the relationship between the therapist and the family has not developed well or is a new one. The data indicates that drastic changes must be accomplished quickly in the parents' behavior in order to mitigate some of the problems developing in the family and also to give the parents a much more effective role in attempting to work with the delinquent. Here it would take a much more directive approach in determining what problem behaviors need to be worked through. The therapist would go directly to those behaviors, discuss them with the parents and offer very specific suggestions as to what changes should be made. In essence, the therapist would be programming the parents to engage in those behaviors deemed necessary to effectively change the relationship between the delinquent and the family. This would be based upon the data that identifies the specific situations in which behavioral interactions lead to very negative kind of repercussions for both members of the family.

Any number of models can be used in working with the parents, from specific role playing techniques to give them the necessary verbal and non-verbal behavior, to the use of a basic shaping procedure on the part of the therapist for the parent's behavior. Here, the specific goal is to allow the parents to create a much greater impact in terms of the on-going family situation and to allow them to exercise all the powerful controls available to them as parents in a significantly more affective and meaningful way than they have apparently been doing in the past.

Here, as in the other situation, the more quickly you can show a successful change in behavior the stronger your position will be in helping the parents to continue to change in the necessary direction. Therefore, in a selection of any of the parents' behavior that you want to change as it relates to the delinquent in the family, the problem selected should be a simple one, a very obvious one, and one that from your professional judgment, will show the greatest degree of change with the suggestions that you are going to institute in the parent-child relationship. One must be cautioned not to select a problem area that will be so long term in treatment and so difficult to change that the degree of frustration that sets in will far exceed the ability to succeed. If necessary the parents and child are to begin to change their own behavior and in this case in the direction of more positive interrelationship.

Other than a recognition, there are a variety of techniques that exist in the field of behavior change, ranging from non-directive therapy to very directive varieties of behavior-modification and behavior therapy. The treatment of choice should be determined by the therapist in conjunction with the family based upon the observations and data collection used in assessing the initial problem.

The literature listed in the bibliography at the end of this chapter make available to the practitioner a wide range of resources and variety of treatment techniques that can be identified and adopted.

The critical issue for the practitioner to be aware of is the variety of treatment programs that exist in the literature far exceed the general range of problems you are likely to encounter in any given situation. What is most critical is the preliminary steps in which an assessment of the particular problem allows you to select the treatment of choice. In the case of working with parents of chronic delinquents, the situations are very similar to any home environment in which the parents find themselves in a position of very little meaningful behavior control, particularly as it relates to the problem child. In this sense, a generalized home management program can be developed, keyed to the range of problems presented by the delinquent in the family putting us in a position to effectively bring about some changes both in the behavior of the delinquent and in the behavior of the parents.

With this concept of the change intervention model, we can now recognize that in many cases two factors will be operating. First is the need to support the parents through their serious trials and tribulations and secondly to significantly alter the behavior of the parent so that they become more effective in working with their delinquent child. Consequently, a combination treatment-support model would use both programs previously discussed.

III. COMBINATION SUPPORT-CHANGE INTERVENTION

The sequence in ordering the intervention would include support first. When this has become an effective intervention then change in the behavior of the parent would come next. Support would never be discontinued, but the focus would move from support to behavior change. The degree to which the parents effectively are able to change their behavior and consequently effectively change the behavior of their delinquent child, will determine the need for support. It is expected it will become somewhat less, because the parents will begin to have successes that they themselves can look to and allow themselves a good degree of self-reinforcement and self-support.

Ultimately, the goal of any intervention with the child and with the parents is to give the necessary maintenance and controls of that behavior to those who must exist in the situation. Therefore, the degree to which the parents can begin to become self-supportive, capable of determining the situation and the appropriate behaviors for their situation on their own, is where the therapist has been singly effective in carrying out their role in altering the problem.

Just as the therapist must determine and assess the nature of the behavior problem, this is also something that the parent must be taught by the therapist to allow them to more fully appreciate what is happening within the situation that is producing the greatest degree of stress, and to allow them to focus on those areas with the most meaningful attempts at behavior change.

To summarize, there are a number of basic steps necessary for a practitioner to follow to be most effective in working with the parents of chronic delinquent youths. First, is a critical need to observe and assess the nature of the parent-child interactions. This includes not only interviews and observations of the parent in the office but through home visitations and discussions with those who have input into the family situation so that a comprehensive picture can be developed of what conditions are and how things exist in the day-to-day life of the parent and the delinquent youth.

Second, based upon these observations, the practitioner must decide what mode of therapy is most desirable. First, we discussed a supportive type, in which the stress on the parents is shared to some degree by the therapist to allow them to function more capably under the conditions that exist, to allow them to have access to a resource on a continual basis in helping them understand the nature of the situation and to feel free to call on somebody when questions come up or when they feel that they are in some kind of crisis situation.

We have pointed out that in a chronic delinquency situation the frequency of the problems are going to be very high, the duration of the stress situations are going to be quite long and a supportive role on the part of the therapist becomes critically important.

We talked about a change intervention role in which the therapist determines from his observations of the problem that the parents are themselves functioning ineffectively and very basic behavior changes are necessary on their part for them to begin to have a positive interaction with the delinquent. The parents are shown, either through directed changes in their behavior, through a process of shaping their behavior, or through a combination of insight and alternative presentations of behavior, what they can now do to change the relationship between them and the delinquent. Here the stress is on selecting a problem area that has a high likelihood of successful change, so that the parents of the child can taste success early rather than continually building up another frustration that has become part of the chronicity of the problem.

Finally, we talked about a combination role in which the therapist would find himself both giving support, particularly during the early stages of the relationship with the family, and then initiating a combination support-behavior change model in which work with the parent would be to find alternative behaviors to the ones they are using, while at the same time giving them strong support for the crisis situations that occur. The focus and goal of all the situations are to allow the parent to become self-supportive, to allow them to become able to modify and adjust their own behavior to handle situations, and to produce a significant change within the complex of the family situation as it relates to the parents and the delinquent child.

In closing, let me again reiterate that techniques for behavior change are available in a variety of journals and in a variety of books which are cited at the end of this chapter. What is often missing is the ability to determine what is the treatment of choice for the given problem that one is facing. With the recognition of the need to work in the home if we are to effectively change the behavior of the problem child, we should realize that in working in the home we are talking specifically about working with the parents. A necessary factor in working in a situation where the problem is chronic delinquency is to assess through observation and data collection what are the problems that the parents themselves have and what the problems are as the parents relate to the delinquent child. From this gathering of data and assessment of the situation, one is in a better position to determine what is the treatment of choice and what intervention should be done. It would be expected that the degree of successful outcome is far better for this kind of preparation than it would be if one were to simply get involved in a situation without determining what all the variables were that were part of the relationship between the parents and the chronic delinquent.

One additional note that can be very helpful for all concerned. Clarification of the roles and responsibilities of the parents and the therapist are very important. In order to measure the degree of accountability assumed by all concerned, a contract between the therapist and the family in which all the particulars are spelled out can be a very valuable tool for treatment and determining the degree of success. This should be entered and modified as the therapist's involvement with the parents changes. It will serve as an excellent guideline for the behavior of all concerned.

REFERENCES

Aldrich, C. K.: Thief. *Psychol Today*, 4:10, 1971.

Bailey, Jon S., Wolf, M. M., and Philips, E. L.: Home-based reinforcement and the modification of pre-delinquent's classroom behavior. *J Appl Behav Anal*, 3:5, 1970.

Bandura, A.: *Principles of Behavior Modification*. New York, Holt, Rinehart, and Winston, 1969.

Becher, W. C.: *Parents Are Teachers: A Child Management Program*. Research Press, 1971.

Bijou, S. W. and Baer, D. M.: *Child Development: Readings in Environmental Analysis*. New York, Appleton, 1967.

Burchard, J., and Tyler, V., Jr.: The modification of delinquent behavior through operant conditioning. *Behav Res Ther*, 2:245-250, 1965.

Coe, W. C.: *A Family Operant Program*. Paper presented at Western Psychological Association, Los Angeles, 1970.

Deibert, A. N., and Harmon, A. V.: *New Tools for Changing Behavior*. Research Press, 1970.

Engela, R., Kawtson, J., Laughy, L., and Garlington, W.: Behavior modification techniques applied to a family unit—A case study, *J Child Psychol Psychiatry*, 9:245-252, 1968.

Guerney, B. F., Jr. (Ed.): *Psychotherapeutic Agents: New Roles for Non-Professionals, Parents, and Teachers*. New York, Holt, Rinehart, and Winston, Inc., 1969.

Hall, R. U.: *Managing Behavior*. Part I Behavior Modification—The Measurement of Behavior; Part II Behavior Modification—Basic Principles; Part III Behavior Modification-Application in School and Home. H & E Enterprises, Inc., 1970.

Hawkins, R. P., Peterson, R. F., Schevard, Edda, and Byere, S. W.: Behavior therapy in the home: Amelioration of problem parent-child relations with the parent in a therapeutic role. *J Exp Child Psychol 4*:99-107, 1966.

Holland, C. J.: An interview guide for behavioral counseling with parents. *Behav Ther 1*:70-79, 1970.

Johnson, James M.: *Using Parents as Contingency Managers.* Paper presented at Eastern Psychological Association, 1969.

Johnson, S. M., and Brown, R. A.: Producing behavior change in parents of disturbed children. *J Child Psychol Psychiatry, 10*:107-121, 1969.

Krumboltz, J. D., and Thoresen, C. E.: *Behavioral Counseling: Cases and Techniques.* New York, Holt, Rinehart, and Winston, 1969.

McIntire, R. W.: *For Love of Children: Behavioral Psychology for Parents.* Del Mar, Calif., C. R. M. Books, 1970.

McIntire, Roger W.: Spare the rod, use behavior mod. *Psychol Today, 4*:1, 1970.

Mira, M.: Results of a behavior modification training program for parents and teachers. *Behav Res Ther, 8*:309-311, 1970.

Patterson, G. R., and Ebner, M. J.: *Applications of Learning Principle to the Treatment of Deviant Children.* American Psychological Association Convention, Chicago, 1965.

Patterson, G. R., and Fagot, B. I.: Selective responsiveness to social reinforcers and deviant behavior in children. *Psychol Record, 17*:369-378, 1967.

Patterson, G. R., Littman, R. E., and Hinsey, W. C.: Parental effectiveness as reinforcers in the laboratory and its relation to child rearing practices and child adjustment in the classroom. *J Pers, 32*:180-199, 1964.

Peine, H. A.: *Programming the Home.* Paper presented to Rocky Mountain Psychological Association, 1969.

Ray, R. S.: *Parents and Teachers as Therapeutic Agents in Behavior Modification.* Paper presented to Second Annual Alabama Behavior Modification Institute, 1969.

Rickard, H. C. (Ed.): *Behavioral Intervention in Human Problems.* Elmsford, N. Y., Pergamon, 1972.

Schwitzgebel, R. L.: Short-term operant conditioning of adolescent offenders on socially relevant variables. *J Abnorm Psychol, 72*:137-142, 1967.

Shala, S. A.: *Training and Utilizing a Mother as a Therapist for Her Child.* Paper presented to Eastern Psychological Association, 1967.

Stuart, R. B.: *Behavioral Contracting Within the Families of Delinquents.* Paper presented at American Psychological Association, 1970.

Tharp, R. G., and Wetzel, R. J.: *Behavior Modification in the Natural Environment.* New York Acad Pr, 1969.

Thorne, G., Tharp, R., and Wetzel, R.: Behavior modification techniques: New tools for probation officers. *Fed Probation* (March, 1967).

Terdal, L., and Buell, J.: Parent education in managing retarded children with behavior deficits and inappropriate behaviors. *Ment Retard, 7:* no. 3, 10-13, 1969.

Tighe, T. J., and Elliott, R.: A technique for controlling behavior in natural life settings. *J Appl Behav Anal, 1:* no. 3, 263-266, 1968.

Ulrich, R., Stachaik, T., and Mabry, J.: *Control of Human Behavior: From Cure to Prevention.* Glenview, Ill. Scott F 1970.

Wagner, M. K.: Parent therapists: An operant conditioning method. *Ment Hyg, 52:452-455,* 1968.

Walder, L. O., Cohen, S. J., Breiter, D. W., Warman, F. C., Orme-Johnson, D., and Pauey, S.: Parents As Change Agents. In Golann, S. E., and Eisdorfer, C. (Eds.): *Handbook of Community Psychology.* New York, Appleton, 1971.

Wahler, R. G., Winkel, G., Peterson, R., and Morrison, D.: Mothers as behavior therapists for their own children. *Behav Res Ther, 3:113-124,* 1965.

Chapter VIII

PSYCHOLOGICAL MANAGEMENT OF THE FAMILY AND THE DYING CHILD

David A. Vore and Logan Wright

- ■ The Child
- ■ The Family
- ■ Technical Considerations
- ■ Conclusion

DESPITE THE INFINITE COMPLEXITIES of individual differences, there are two experiences which everyone must undergo—birth and death. These experiences signify the beginning of the developmental process in the external environment and the end of that same process. Although faced with the fact that death will at some time be experienced by each and every individual, psychology has, for some reason, ignored or avoided seriously looking at the process and attempting to understand its emotional impact upon people. Only recently have clinicians such as Elisabeth Kubler-Ross (1969), Avery Weisman (1972), William M. Easson (1970), and others dealt with the process of dying and its emotional impact upon the individual. With the acknowledgement of the existence of death and the gradually increasing awareness of the emotional sequelae to it has come an increase in the number of clinicians attempting to deal with the problem. The purpose of this particular chapter is to aid the professional who chooses to work with the problem of the dying child and his family.

This paper will focus on management of the dying child and

his family and will be "practitioner oriented" in the sense that it will not be a literature review or a philosophical treatise on the problem. However, our purpose in writing the chapter is not to present a formula or cookbook approach which can be followed by the clinician as he deals with these kinds of problems. It is, rather, to present the major concerns and problem areas encountered in attempting to work with these patients in a manner which will be meaningful to the practitioner. The information presented is based upon our own experiences in working with terminally ill children and their families in the Department of Pediatrics, Children's Memorial Hospital, an affiliate of the University of Oklahoma Health Sciences Center. The chapter will focus on the child suffering from leukemia or other types of cancer. However, it is felt that the principles discussed are applicable to children experiencing other types of terminal illness.

The remainder of the paper will be divided into three major sections. The first of these will deal with the understanding and management of the terminally ill child himself. The typical stages a child goes through in his conceptualization of death, the needs typically expressed by the terminally ill child and the approach we have found to be most productive will be focussed upon. The second section will deal with the management of the family of the dying child. Needs of the various members of the family, questions asked by family members, the types of crises most commonly encountered by the family of the dying child, the stages of acceptance and some common dynamic issues will be discussed. In addition, examples will be given of the types of severe pathology which are sometimes precipitated in family members by the occurrence of terminal illness in a child. The third section will be directed toward examination of the various techniques which can be used with both the terminally ill child himself and family members.

THE CHILD

The child who suffers from a terminal illness such as leukemia or a type of solid tumor may be referred to a psychologist for a variety of reasons. These reasons are, of course, as varied as the number of children who are referred. However, four major issues do seem to occur rather consistently which are usually expressed in questions about whether to tell a child about his disease, how to tell him, how to manage behavioral problems, and how to best support the child. These four questions can best be exemplified through a presentation of a hypothetical referral request.

T. J. is a seven-year-old male who has recently been diagnosed as having acute lymphoblastic leukemia. The diagnosis was made in a separate clinical facility and the parents and child were referred to our clinic for treatment and management of the course of the disease. During the initial interview with the parents, they both expressed great concern and grief over their son's diagnosis. In addition, they very emphatically stated that T. has not yet been told of his disease nor will be ever be told as long as they have anything to say about it. When asked for the reasons behind this, both parents flatly state that they simply feel there is no reason for T. to worry and become upset over "what he has." This type of situation is a common one and, in fact, will often arise even when a child is seen for an initial diagnosis in our own clinic. The common factor which seems to underlie all such problems is the need of the parents themselves to deny awareness or acknowledgement of the disease process currently active in their child and its ultimate outcome. Consequently, they refuse to grapple with the problem themselves, and, in so doing, refuse to allow the child the opportunity to come to grips with his disease and its meaning for him. What generally develops, then, is an unagreed upon but, nevertheless, very effective "pact of silence" between the parents and the child and a refusal to communicate about the disease.

One of the most unfortunate consequences of such a situation involves the plight of the child patient. In this case, T. is faced with a number of things. First of all, he will be hospitalized for a period of days and possibly weeks in order to start him on a given treatment protocol. During the hospitalization he will be faced with IV procedures, bone marrows, blood samples, and so on. In addition, depending upon the course of chemotherapy chosen, he is likely to experience a variety of side effects from whatever medication is used ranging from transitory pains in his extremities through nausea, mouth ulcers and loss of hair. He will be constantly besieged by a variety of nursing personnel, medical students, house staff, and others. Upon his discharge from the hospital, he will be allowed to go home, but he will feel weak and will find it takes him some time to regain his old level of stamina. In addition, he will be asked to return to the hospital on a regular basis for monitoring of his disease process and the treatment program. Even though his disease may be temporarily arrested (remission), he will still be periodically administered bone marrows as part of his regular treatment program. Following this apparent improvement the leukemia will most likely return (relapse) and he will again be admitted to the hospital where he will undergo basically the same procedure as previously described. The process of remission and relapse may occur many times during the course of treatment. In addition, the child will be subjected to a variety of situations where adults (parents, friends, physicians, etc.) talk about him in hushed tones, and he will in some cases overhear their remarks. Given this situation, it is hard to imagine any child who will not ask the question of "what is wrong with me" and, further, who does not begin to view himself as being critically ill. The point of all this is simply that whether the child knows the actual label assigned to his disease, whether or not he knows beyond a shadow of a doubt that he will probably die as a result of the disease, we are of the opinion that he certainly gradually becomes aware of the fact that he is a special child and that his degree of speciality is dictated by the fact that he is very sick. He may have a number of questions which he wants to ask concerning his disease but he will be unable to find answers because of his conspiracy of silence with his parents. The position that such a child is in is one of learning that important people in his environment, primarily his parents, do not want to talk about this "terrible thing he has" and that only pained looks and, at best, clumsy, half true answers will follow questions about the matter. In time, he also begins to feel that he must protect his parents and other family members from himself by denying his disease process. The message he is being given by them indicates this to be what they want. Thus, on top of not feeling well and experiencing anxiety about his disease, he is also forced to deny it and to essentially protect others at the cost of not coming to grips with his disease and its meaning for himself.

One common consequence of this process involves the development of antagonism between parents who don't want their child told about his disease, and the medical staff treating their child who feel he must be told. In such cases we have found that the best approach consists of two steps. First, the parents must learn to acknowledge their child's disease and to work through their grief, anxiety, and other feelings about it. It is not until they have reached a stage of at least partial acceptance themselves that they can begin to provide the support for the child which he so badly needs. The second step, which by no means must necessarily come after the work just described with the parents, involves working with the medical staff with the goal of helping them understand their probable anger and frustration with parents who will not allow them to "clear their conscience" by informing the child about his disease.

Once the clinician has completed or perhaps gotten well into the two processes just described, he can then work with, and hopefully through, the parents to accomplish the goal of at least beginning communication with the child about his disease. The underlying assumption, of course, is that the child has a need and most certainly a right to come to grips with his disease and its probable outcome to the best of his ability.

At this time, the second question is generally asked of how to tell the child whatever it is that his parents and the medical staff have decided that he should know. The fear that most parents express at this point is that they will be asked to simply walk in, sit down with their child and state, "T., you have leukemia and you are probably going to die from it." Their second fear is that even if they are not forced to do this, someone else will do it for them. Our response to this is generally as follows. "It is important that the child be allowed to deal with his disease on his own terms and at the level at which he is capable of functioning." Thus, there is probably no need to approach a child in the

way parents fear he will be approached. Rather, what the parent
or the psychologist must do is provide the child a warm, supporting, caring, and open individual with whom to talk and share
questions, fantasies, etc. In many cases, it is necessary to help the
child along by providing some type of stimulation such as asking
him to draw pictures or, perhaps, observing him in a play situation. At no time is the goal to force the child to deal with his
disease at the same level of awareness or the same level of understanding as the adult deals with it. The task is to move at the
child's speed and to relate to the child on his own level.

A number of people have addressed themselves to the stages
of awareness of death which the child goes through as he progresses along the developmental path. In our experience, we have
found a combination of the conceptualization presented by Dr.
Kubler-Ross (1972) and the developmental approach of Erik
Erikson (1964) to be the most useful one in dealing with children.

The very young child (six months to two years) without question perceives and responds to concerns, fears, and anxiety of
significant others in his environment. However, he basically lacks
the communication skills necessary to verbally label his fears or
concerns and he cannot, therefore, enter into a significant verbal
communication concerning them. Essentially, then, in the very
young child, although we never really know his view of death,
it would seem that the major response to serious illness hinges
around the discomfort caused and the failure of significant others (parents) in his environment to make the hurt go away and
allow him to feel comfortable, satisfied, and fulfilled again. In
many respects this stage of dealing with death is probably most
akin to concepts which have been presented by Erikson when he
specified the stage of "basic trust" as being the first stage of ego
development in the child's developmental sequence. That is, the
infant is completely dependent upon parents for satisfaction of
needs such as hunger, warmth, and shelter. The infant responds
in terms of the loss of these satisfactions on a momentary basis.
Losing comfort is important in an equilibration sense, in that
the infant, of course, wishes to have the comfort restored. How-

ever, he is completely dependent upon some other force in his environment to do so. If comfort is not restored, the loss experienced by the organism is in terms of this momentary comfort state and frustration arises resulting from the failure of significant others to restore it. Experientially, then, there is probably no concept of death, and therefore, no fear of dying as we know it in the child at this age. Instead, there is a "fear" of a reaction to loss of comfort which the infant must depend upon parents to provide.

As the child grows older, approximately two years to four years of age, he moves from the stage of "basic trust" to one of "autonomy" according to Erikson's scheme. During this time, he is beginning to differentiate the "me" from the "not me" in his environment. He becomes ruled by the desire to determine how effective his own behavior is upon manipulating the environment. In addition, the child attempts to avoid being controlled by elements in his environment and consequently enters into the period often referred to by parents as "the terrible two's and terrible three's." During this period of ego development, the child may begin to develop the beginnings of a concept of death. Typically, however, at this time death is primarily associated with separation from important others. The child is now able to distinguish himself from the other important individuals in his environment, at least on a very elementary level. In addition, he is striving mightily to develop an independence and freedom from those others. However, his behavior is also characterized by tentative returns to the comfort of these important people. During this time, then, the major feeling the child has concerning death focuses on his anticipation and fear of losing things and people which he has differentiated from himself but which he is still to a certain extent dependent upon and which he still needs. Thus, children at this age who talk about death do so in terms of questions and statements such as "if I die will I have my dog with me?, where is Grandpa since he's died—can he see us—is Grandma with him; when Bobby dies and goes to heaven who will help him to take a bath?" The major fear and fantasy of children at this age concerns being shut away and separated from anything and everything which is important to them and never again being able to establish contact with these things.

Between the ages of, roughly, four and six, the child enters into the stage labeled by Erikson as the "initiative stage." This stage is also occasionally referred to as the "intrusion or intrusive period." During this stage the child is rapidly discovering the myriad possibilities which the world has to offer. He becomes extremely assertive and aggressive in his exploratory attempts and, in addition, begins to become quite demanding in terms of interactions with others. In his attempts to force interaction and gain attention, he is beginning to develop a concept of himself as important and worthy of attention levied by others. However, he is also, typically, experiencing considerable rejection (unfortunately) and punishment due to the intrusive nature of his interactions. At the same time, as Dr. Kubler-Ross points out, he is beginning to make forays into the outside world and, as he wanders, he may become acutely aware of the presence of death in animals which have been struck by cars or otherwise physically mangled. Thus, his immediate concept of death has to do with being mangled, crushed or in some other fashion mutilated by an extremely powerful and probably capricious force in the environment. In addition, in most cases this force has something to do with adults who generally seem to be all-knowing and all-powerful. At this time, then, the child's view of death largely becomes one of punishment and mutilation. That is, death is obviously something which leaves a bleeding and crushed body behind. In addition, when one transgresses or in some fashion causes displeasure of powerful others in the environment, one is rewarded with a spanking or some other form of punishment. Who is to say, then, that the ultimate punishment is not to be made very sick, to be forced to endure bone marrows, shots, and other unpleasantness, and finally to die for having caused the displeasure of parents.

Between the years of approximately seven and the beginning of adolescence, the child is progressing through the stage labeled by Erikson as "industry." Basically, during this stage the child is developing a self-concept of success, and of being in control over things that happen to him, at least to some extent. In addition, Jean Piaget (1969) has also indicated that during this period the child is progressing in terms of cognitive development so that he has a clear understanding of time dimensions as well as the ability to reason in a logical fashion, which allows him to understand the difference between "being and not being." In terms of the conception of death, the most significant characteristic of the child during these years seems to be the development of the aspect of permanence to the state of death. Much of the child's experience during his early years consists of viewing death on television or reading about it in books. He views it as being something which happens but which (1) won't happen to him, and (2) which he never really grapples with in terms of the concept of permanence. So it is, at this time, that brothers and sisters of the terminally ill child tells stories and relate great affect over the fact that when Billy dies he will never come back and they will never see him again. In addition, it is also during this period that the terminally ill child himself begins to make statements such as "don't cry mommy, I will be alright" with no implication that there will be a reunion or reuniting at some time in the future.

From the beginning of the adolescent years the individual goes through two more stages which have been labeled by Erikson to be "identity" and "intimacy." It is during this time that the adolescent is beginning to develop a true conception of himself for what he is. That is, he is beginning to define himself as attractive or unattractive, strong or weak, effective or ineffective, desirable or undesirable, etc. In addition, he is beginning to develop very strong relationships with both members of the same sex and of the opposite sex. In fact, he begins to define his worth to some extent in terms of his success in achieving this kind of imtimacy. The adolescent with a terminal illness, then, is outraged at the unfairness of his illness. He deeply resents his loss of independence in terms of being told when to come back to the hospital, what medicines to take or how to conduct his life. He has an extremely difficult time maintaining a positive self-image in terms of being attractive, successful, and effective since he often does not feel well, he is "disfigured" through the loss of hair or the development of facial blemishes, and he loses the energy to successfully take on and dominate his environment. He may often become deeply depressed, uncommunicative, or withdrawn and may simply refuse to follow the treatment program prescribed for him. In addition, he may refuse to allow his family to comfort him and, as is the case with the younger child, often finds himself in a position of having to deny his disease in order to "protect his family." Basically, the stages of dealing with the terminal illness which an adolescent goes through are the same as those described by Dr. Elisabeth Kubler-Ross (1969) based on her work with terminally ill adults. The primary difference, perhaps, lies in the extreme anger which the adolescent feels with respect to his loss of independence and freedom.

The question, therefore, is not *whether* to tell a child that he has a terminal illness, but how to tell him. The answer to this question lies in the realization that children do seem to go through rather definite developmental steps in their concept of death. As they progress through these various stages, the fantasies which they experience and the questions which they ask will vary. The task of the clinician or parent dealing with the child who has a terminal illness is not to attempt to force his own level of awareness and understanding upon the child, but, rather, to allow him to deal with the problem at his own speed and at his own level. If a child expresses fear of mutilation and punishment, this must be accepted and then assurance given that such is not the case.

The third type of question which often confronts the clinician working with the dying child and his family has to do with problems of management. Essentially, the feeling that most parents go through is one of total frustration and inability to contribute in any meaningful way to the treatment of the child's illness and to his possible return to health. This feeling, in combination with feelings of guilt (which will be dealt with at a later point in this chapter) and a general feeling of pity for the child often lead to a situation where one or both parents are totally ineffective in managing the sick child and perhaps siblings as well. The kinds of questions which come up are usually ones such as "why should I discipline Billy when I know he is already in so much pain; I know I am easier with Suzy than with my other children but I just can't bring myself to discipline her; etc." In some cases we have found ourselves to be dealing with parents who lacked basic management skills prior to the child's illness. However, in an equally large number of cases, we are faced with parents who were effective prior to the child's illness but who find themselves ineffective in the face of the child's disease. What has actually happened is that the parent or parents are finding themselves totally disarmed in terms of their rationale for and comfort with the usual management skills which are effective with children.

The approach we take in such cases is two-fold. First of all, it is necessary to deal with the feelings of despair, guilt, and frustration which the parents feel. Second, we enter into what is essentially a parent skills training sequence with, ideally, both parents of any given child. These sessions focus on the need that every child has for discipline and for structure set by his parents. In addition, we generally find it necessary and productive to discuss various techniques which the parents might try with the child as well as with sibs. We encourage them to return to their family situation with the goal of trying a variety of approaches and discussing their effectiveness and/or problems with us. The parental response to such an approach has been overwhelmingly positive.

If a child is old enough, we often work with him or her directly in terms of the management problems. That is, an attempt is made to help the child understand his manipulativeness and the gain which occurs from it. In many cases a child will begin to "use" his disease as a way of manipulating parents and others in his environment. This is a typical response and is one which must be taken on directly in order to reduce stress on the family system. The child's anger, fear and frustration which lead to his demands for demonstration from others that he is cared for and loved must be labeled and dealt with. In addition, the child's reactions to the structure placed upon him by his parents and by others in his environment must also be considered.

The fourth major issue as far as the child himself is concerned has to do with the position which he is often forced to occupy with respect to his parents and significant others in his environment. The terminally ill child is usually faced with a fairly long series of treatments which are often painful and which are certainly frightening to the child. He is at a time in his life when, perhaps more than at any other time, he needs the support, love, and understanding of his parents and of those with whom he is in contact. In many cases, however, we have found the child to be placed in exactly the opposite role. That is, because the parents themselves (and often ward staff and/or the treatment team as well) seem to be unable to deal with the crisis and continually send messages that they do not want to be confronted with it, particularly in his presence, the child finds himself forced into a position of having to protect and support those who should be supporting him. He is, thus, forced to not talk about his illness, not express his fears, not ask questions which are of tremendous importance to him because he does not want to force parents and others into the unpleasant situation of having to acknowledge and deal with his illness. This is particularly true of the older child and of the early adolescent. The result, predictably, of such a role definition for the child is an environment which forces denial and consequently lack of acceptance of all that is happening. A frequent concomitant of this denial is anger and frustration on the part of the child which is expressed in a passive-aggressive manner towards the parents. Hence, referrals are made for problems such as management difficulties referred to above, depression, withdrawal, and so on.

The clinician faced with such a situation has two choices. First of all, he can attempt to deal with the parents and make them aware of what is happening with the child. However, their ability to reverse their behavior depends upon their ability to work through their own feelings and acceptance of the disease process in their child. This may take a considerable amount of time and it is therefore often necessary for the clinician himself to provide the child with an opportunity to deal with his disease. In doing this the clinician cannot, obviously, simply walk into a child's room and say "tell me about your disease" or "tell me about your feelings about death." What he must do is establish a warm, trusting, open relationship with the child and be extremely sensitive to symbolic communications from the child. These may take the form of verbal, or non-verbal communications such as tears, withdrawal, drawings or stories. The task of the clinician is to be sensitive to these communications and to respond to them in a manner which will allow the child to more fully explore the feeling underlying them.

THE FAMILY

In discussing the family of the dying child, the first concern must be the parents of the child, since in practically every case the clinician will be called upon to work with them. In our experience with parents, we have found that they tend to go through a fairly well-defined and circumscribed series of stages in their attempts to deal with the tragedy which has befallen their child and themselves. This in no way implies that each and every parent will go through each and every stage in the same manner or at the same rate. It simply indicates that the typical progression of dealing with the issue of death in a child tends to follow a very well-defined sequence. Dr. Elisabeth Kubler-Ross (1969) has written extensively on the dying patient and the stages which the adult usually goes through as he attempts to deal with his own terminal illness. She has indicated (Kubler-Ross, 1972), and we have also found, that parents of dying children also seem to go through these same stages. We feel it will be useful to discuss each of these stages with respect to the typical kinds of problems that seem to be associated with them for most parents. In addition, we feel it necessary to point out that one major thing which we have learned in dealing with parents of the terminally ill child has been that one must not strip defenses away from the individual. If and when the parent is ready to give up a defense and progress to another stage, he or she will let the clinician know in some manner.

The initial reaction of parents to diagnosis of a terminal illness in a child is one of shock and a sense of being overwhelmed by the diagnosis and its implications. This is followed by denial of both the disease and its probable outcome. Many parents will state that they understand that "Johnny has leukemia" but they will hasten to add that they know that in some cases leukemia has been cured. They then follow this up with a statement to the effect that they are confident that their child *will* be cured. Using this type of statement and the rationalization of the great advances being made in medicine every day, the parent is able to completely avoid or deny the disease and he certainly never allows himself to think or speak of the possibility of death occurring. Most parents will defend their stance at this time by indicating that they feel that they must have hope and by asking the question of why the development of hope is not adaptive. The problem is that this type of hope is part of a stronger denial of the reality of the situation. That is, this hope supports the parent in his refusal to hear and understand the true situation facing the child. If the parent is unable to ever move past this particular point of denial, one of two things will usually happen. At the time that the child does in fact die, the parent will be completely unprepared for it and may go into a profound depression. The other consequence is seen in the parent who begins to attempt to support his denial by any and every means available to him. One of the most common means available is to shut the child out in an experiential sense. That is, the parent withdraws emotional ties and emotional contact from the child in an effort to avoid being faced with any kind of situation which may challenge or contradict the very strong denial system which he or she has constructed.

The clinician attempting to deal with denial must recognize that, to some extent, it is encountered in all of us when we attempt to deal with the concept of death, either our own or that of someone very close to us. It is only when this defense completely takes over and when the individual's behavior is totally based on the denial that it becomes a major problem. When this is the case we have found that the best way to approach the parent is not to directly confront them with what they are doing, since this usually results in an increased effort to maintain the denial, but rather to provide them with support and empathy and an understanding of the need which they feel to avoid dealing with the tragedy of their child's impending death. In most cases, if the clinician is successful in providing this type of climate, the parent will eventually be able to give up the denial, at least in the extreme form which has been described.

The second stage a parent seems to go through is that of anger. The anger may be expressed in overt or passive aggressive ways toward medical staff, siblings of the terminally ill child, the other parent, or the child himself. Often the expression of the anger will take the form of strong criticism of the treatment being offered the child, the lack of concern expressed by others toward the child or refusal to follow the therapy program which is prescribed. We have found two major factors which seem to be associated with the development of this anger. The first of these has to do with the tremendous frustration which a parent feels. The frustration is largely focussed on the fact that the parent loves, wants to support, and wants to be needed by the child. However, particularly during the times when the child is in the hospital, the parent is given a very clear message that the medical staff can and will do any and everything possible to cure the child. Thus the parent is forced to grapple with the fact that what happens to the child, at least in terms of survival or maintenance of health, is completely out of his or her hands. One very typical reaction to this is to demonstrate to others that in fact he, as parent, is not powerless and that he can have some say in what happens to the child even to the extent of thwarting the efforts made by the medical team. Another type of frustration seems to revolve around the question of "why us." The parent must grapple with the experience of looking at other children or looking at other parents who don't seem to care for their children and, yet, have healthy, normal offspring. The inability to answer the question "why" is highly tension-producing and also results in a very strong feeling of frustration.

The second factor associated with the anger is often found

to be very strong feelings of guilt. It is not unusual for a parent to feel that the child's illness is a function of some deficit in his own genetic make-up. In these cases no amount of counseling by a medical person with respect to the nongenetic basis of leukemia or cancer seems to have an impact upon the parent. Thus, a mother can state very clearly "I know that my child is not dying because of some genetic weakness in me. But, I also perceive myself as a frail, fragile person and I strongly feel that if he had another mother he would not be sick." A similar guilt is found in the parent who feels he or she is being punished for some transgression, real or imagined, which was performed in the past. The behavioral effects of such a feeling will be examined in the discussion of the third stage of acceptance.

Another facet of guilt is expressed by the parent who makes the statement "Billy had been complaining for several weeks, and I thought all along that he was just being babyish." These parents are faced with the fear that had they listened and responded to their child's complaints earlier they might have been able to obtain treatment for him which would have come soon enough to save his life. Again, no amount of counseling by a medical person with respect to the reality of such a statement seems to have much effect. What is necessary in dealing with this type of guilt is to aid the parent in expressing it, labeling it and understanding that although the feeling is there, it is not a reality based fear.

The guilt and frustration which the parent faces often leads to the development of strong anger which is very difficult for the parent to deal with. A typical statement which might be made by a parent working through this aspect of the impending death of their child would be something to the effect of "I guess I am mad, but there's no one for me really to be angry at." That is, a parent cannot express anger toward the child, their mate or their God. There seems to be no one or nothing to which they can point and say "It's your fault and you are bad and evil." Consequently, the anger generally comes out in the more indirect and passive-aggressive ways previously mentioned.

As a parent works through the denial and becomes aware of

the anger, he begins to phase into a third stage which has been labeled the "bargaining stage." At this point the parent is no longer as effectively denying that his or her child is seriously ill nor is he denying the probability of death as the outcome of the disease. In addition, he is beginning to become aware of some of his own feelings and responses to the disease and with this awareness he reaches a stage where he begins to feel that if he understands and accepts everything and behaves in just the optimal manner, that perhaps the child's illness will be conquered and he will get well. In its own way this is another form of denial on the part of the parent. However, it is also an attempt by the parent to assume some responsibility and some role in the ultimate outcome of the course of his child's disease. That is, he begins to view himself as being a key figure in the potential recovery of the child. His role will be to think or act in a manner which will effect the outcome of the child's disease. It is often at this stage that the element of religion seems to play the strongest role. The parent may turn to the Will of God as an explanation for the child's disease and he may further try to justify the Will of God as being a function of some transgression or weakness on his part. Consequently, he feels that if he eliminates the weakness and lives a life which is defined as a "good life," his God will intervene and alter the outcome of the child's disease. This is a particularly difficult stage for the clinician to deal with. We have found that individuals who seem to have a true and basic religion are able to use it effectively in dealing with their child's illness and ultimate death. However, those who seem to turn desperately to religion as an answer usually find it unsuccessful in helping them deal with the disease and they will generally give up this particular "defense" on their own accord.

The fourth stage that a parent goes through is that of depression. At the point where the parent can no longer maintain denial, feelings of being overwhelmed and of despair generally surface. At this point, the parent may express a fear of the desire to give up and get the whole thing over with. Often underlying such feelings, one again finds very strong anger which has been directed inward and of which the parent is generally completely unaware. The anger may often take the form of resentment at the disease and, consequently, at the child for interfering with the life of the parent and of the family. In addition, there is resentment about financial burdens and the complete disruption of family life. The parent will find himself faced with the feeling of "I wish he would die and get it over with, I'm tired of all of this." This is, of course, an extremely painful thing for a parent to feel and there is considerable guilt and need to punish oneself if one allows it into awareness. At this point, a parent especially needs a clinician who is able and willing to fill the role of therapist. The depression must be accepted, the basis of it must be understood and labeled, the parent must be made aware that the feelings are not evil but are perfectly understandable.

The final stage seen in a parent attempting to deal with the terminally ill child is that of acceptance. At the point of acceptance, a parent is able to be fully aware and accepting of the child's illness and its probable ultimate outcome. In addition, the parent is equally aware and accepting of his own reactions and responses to that situation. While anger may exist, the parent is not consumed with guilt, while hope may exist the parent does not use it as a way of hiding from reality. It is at this point that a parent finds himself able to begin to truly deal with questions such as management of the child and of his siblings. In addition, it is at this point that the parent begins to be able to go through a stage or a process of preparatory grieving. During this process, the parent allows himself to feel the impending loss and what it will mean to him. He does not, however, react to this by shutting the child out or by avoiding the situation. It is at this time that a parent can state "I've got to get my grieving done because there is going to be so much to do in the future."

Having taken a look at the stages which parents seem to go through as they deal with their terminally ill child, there are two other aspects of dealing with parents on which we need to focus. The first of these has to do with typical roles or typical reactions seen in mothers and fathers of the terminally ill child. What usually happens is that a father finds he can avoid the situation and maintain some denial by immersing himself in his work. As he withdraws, the mother assumes the role of bringing the child to the hospital for both inpatient and outpatient treatments. Essentially, this forces the mother into the position of having to face the disease in its entirety. She cannot deny as effectively as father since she is the one that sees the bone marrows being drawn, the IV's begun, and the pain which the child goes through during the treatments. At this time, mothers will often express strong feelings of loneliness and anger that they are the ones that have to deal with this without support. The interesting thing is that father usually is able to reenter the situation in the final stages of the disease. He does so as a strong, supporting figure. Our assumption is that, were he unable to withdraw as effectively as he does in the beginning stages of the disease, he would probably not be able to fill this role later. However, we find it often necessary to work through the feelings of aloneness, anger and frustration that a mother has with regard to the situation.

The second comment which must be added at this point has to do with the stress associated with diagnosis and treatment of a child's terminal illness on already existing parental pathology. In some cases a parent finds himself completely unable to respond in an adaptive manner to the stress forced upon him by his child's disease. The types of reactions often seen are of either a paranoid nature or an extreme escape response which may take the form of withdrawal into drugs or alcohol or perhaps severe depression. In these instances, the clinician must be able to provide long-term intensive therapy, perhaps even to the point of hospitalization if necessary. In addition, he must be willing to diagnose and label the behavior as severely pathological and recognize that it is not simply a "typical reaction" to the stress of terminal illness in the child.

Of course, other members of the immediate family are also important. Sibs of the terminally ill child will also be affected by and respond to stress engendered by the child's disease. A critical concern with sibs has to do with their own perception of death and with their fantasies concerning the child's illness and impending death. Dynamic factors such as guilt over sibling rivalry and the desire to be rid of the terminally ill child, jealousy and anger at the terminally ill child and the fear of death themselves, perhaps associated with punishment, are all important aspects to which the clinician must be sensitive. In many cases, we have been tempted to overlook siblings of a terminally ill child since we are more immediately faced with the child himself or with his parents. This is particularly true in cases where siblings do not force us to recognize them and attend to them. We have learned that it is the sibling who is apparently a model, who quietly "accepts" his brother or sister's disease and death and who does nothing to really call attention to himself, who is often likely to have problems in the future. It is important that siblings be allowed and encouraged to work through their own feelings and fears as their brother or sister progresses through the course of the disease. It is also important that the siblings be allowed to proceed through a preparatory grief phase just as parents do prior to the child's death. When this is not done, we have found that problems arise weeks, months, and perhaps years following the death of the child. The most extreme example of this is a fourteen-year-old girl whose brother died when he was approximately ten. She and her brother were described as very close and, at the time of his death, she was mildly upset but did not demonstrate any behavior which called strong attention to herself in any manner. However, four years after her brother's death, she is seen with a presenting complaint of severe nightmares, strong anxiety, and a recent hospitalization for "nervous exhaustion." It is this child and others like her who we must not fail to recognize and attempt to deal with prior to their development of symptomatology such as this.

TECHNICAL CONSIDERATIONS

As we have experienced working with a variety of referrals involving the terminally ill child, we have become aware of the existence of and need for a variety of approaches in dealing with these clients. The primary factor which must be considered regardless of the approach taken has to do with the clinician being a full-member of the hematology-oncology team which is treating the child. Full membership is defined as the clinician holding a position within the "core" of the team and having, therefore, equal input into the development of the treatment model. The reasons for this type of role definition are two-fold. First of all, without such a relationship the clinician rapidly becomes an ancillary person to the treatment team. As such, he begins to occupy a position which allows team members to avoid dealing with their patients in the areas described in this paper by foisting the patients off upon him. Thus, he merely becomes a "dumping ground" for the team. In contrast, we feel that a major role which the clinician must perform concerns working with members of the medical team sometimes in a fashion very similar to that taken in working with parents of the terminally ill child. That is, members of the medical team and the ward staff who deal with the terminally ill child and his parents also have feelings about the disease and about the particular child and also respond to the situation on the basis of these feelings. A critical aspect of the clinician's role, therefore, involves his being a model for the team members as well as helping them periodically assess their own feelings with the goal of becoming aware of how these affect their behavior. A second reason for the clinician being a committed member of the treatment team involves the desirability of his immediate and continuing contact with a child and his family from the very first moment that they are seen by the medical team. In this way, the family can relate to the clinician on a regular basis and consequently not be forced to label themselves as having "emotional problems" before seeking assistance.

There are a variety of approaches which can be taken in dealing with the terminally ill child and his family. The child may been seen individually and the parents as a couple. The entire family may be seen together, or groups may be started for both terminally ill children and/or parents of these children. Each of these approaches has a unique value. The choice of approach is largely determined by the time commitment and personal preferences of the clinician. However, it is worth noting that on a number of occasions parents (particularly mothers) have very strongly indicated their desire for a group experience involving other parents of terminally ill children. The reason for this revolves around their apparent feeling of support and understanding gained from others who are undergoing the same type of experience. It is, therefore, worthwhile considering the development of such a group in any setting in which the clinician is working.

CONCLUSION

The purpose of this chapter has been to present a composite picture of the terminally ill child and his family. The types of questions, issues, and problems, which often arise, have been discussed. When initially thinking about the writing of such a chapter, one goal was to specify methods of dealing with these children and their parents. However, as the development of the chapter progressed, a decision was made to focus instead on the attitudes, feelings, etc. of the child and other family members with the purpose being to make the clinician aware of their existence in his patients. It is felt that attempting to elucidate specific techniques and specific manners of responding to these issues in one single chapter would simply be impossible. Consequently, it is hoped that the reader can fit the information provided in this chapter into his own framework and therapy approach. A note of caution seems appropriate, however. There seems to be one primary factor which is important for the clinician who attempts to deal with these types of cases. That factor involves a clinician's own willingness and ability to grapple with the issue of his own lack of immortality and his own concepts about death. Until he has done this, it is extremely difficult for him to give much service to others who are attempting to do it under much more stressful situations. Finally, it should be noted that attempting to work with the terminally ill patient and his family is an emotionally draining and stressful situation for the clinician himself. However, it is also a highly rewarding effort in that clearly observable behavioral changes can be effected through clinical intervention.

REFERENCES

Easson, W. M.: *The Dying Child: The Management of the Child or Adolescent Who Is Dying.* Springfield, Ill., Charles C Thomas, 1970.

Erikson, E.: *Childhood, Youth and Society*. New York, W. W. Norton and Company, 1964.

Kubler-Ross, E.: *On Death and Dying*. New York, Macmillan, 1969.

———: Children and death. In Vore, D. A. (Chm.): *The Dying Child.* Symposium presented at the meeting of the American Psychological Association, Honolulu, September 1972.

Piaget, J., and Inhelder, B.: *The Psychology of the Child*. New York, Basic Books, Inc., 1969.

Weisman, A. D.: *On Dying and Denying: A Psychiatric Study of Terminality*. New York, Behavioral Publications, 1972.

Chapter IX

SEPARATION COUNSELING: A STRUCTURED APPROACH TO MARITAL CRISIS*

MARJORIE KAWIN TOOMIM

- RATIONALE FOR STRUCTURED SEPARATION WITH COUNSELING
- THE SEPARATION STRUCTURE
- SEPARATION COUNSELING
- SUMMARY

MARRIAGE COUNSELORS AND PSYCHOTHERAPISTS are all too familiar with the couple who comes for help stating they must either "make this marriage work or get a divorce." One partner is generally inclined to cling desperately to the marriage, willing to do almost anything to avoid divorce. The other is desirous of the marriage, but tired of trying and sees no way to go but "out." Trial separation is generally not considered a reasonable alternative. The more threatened of the two is usually afraid to let go of the semblance of control available through physical proximity. The other is looking toward complete freedom. Both may have little tolerance for the lack of structure which is implied by separation as opposed to divorce. This chapter presents a fourth alternative, a moderately structured, time-limited period of separation with counseling.

RATIONALE FOR STRUCTURED SEPARATION WITH COUNSELING

Separation counseling is a form of crisis intervention counseling (Parad, 1965). It is a time-limited approach which deals

---

* This is an expanded version of a paper entitled "Structured Separation With Counseling: A therapeutic approach for couples in conflict (Toomim, 1972).

specifically with the immediate crisis of family separation. The purpose of this counseling procedure is to help separating individuals understand their relationship, resolve their conflicts, decide whether their future relationship will be together or apart, and grow through the separation process.

A major assumption on which separation counseling is based is that a meaningful relationship, once established, can never be altogether lost. It can only be changed. In some cases, especially where there are children, separated partners continue to see each other and make decisions together. If they do not continue to have some tangible connection with each other, they nonetheless continue to relate to each other in fantasy, imagination and memory. It is important that the couple work through the separation process carefully and thoroughly so that little unfinished business remains to interfere with their continuing separation-relationship or in new relationships.

The techniques and methods outlined below are of particular value to separating couples, married or unmarried, and to parents and children who are separating. They may be applied by individuals with or without counseling. However, counseling is especially useful for couples having much difficulty separating, for extremely dependent individuals who are limited in emotional freedom, for those who are afraid to risk, and for those subject to severe depression.

The structured separation provides a firm time-space base within which individuals may maximize their freedom to experience and grow. It minimizes the shock of separation. It makes positive use of the separation process as an aid to development so that individuals neither deny their losses nor become victims to the pain. Respect for self and other, trust, choice, courage, honesty, emotional development, and positive growth are inherent in this method.

Conflict-laden couples who choose to separate voluntarily before their discomfort becomes intolerable, gain much from openly and consciously making this choice. Manipulative and punitive maneuvers, such as capricious sexual behavior, designed to force a break in the relationship are avoided. Such maneuvers often cause irreparable damage, shatter trust, and humiliate one or both mates. In separating voluntarily, the partners signify that each values himself, the other, and what they have between them enough to allow some distance. Such distance provides each with an opportunity to gain perspective and to try alternative solutions to problems. The couple may then come together again with renewed understanding and feeling, or go on to other relationships having learned a great deal from this one. Separation counseling insures that little unfinished business remains to interfere with new experiences.

Structured separation is an excellent model for distressed families with children. These children are thus presented with parental behavior where honesty, choice, and respect are primary values. Some of the damage done by the suddenness and emotional uproar common in most divorce is mitigated. The children have both time and an open interpersonal situation in which to adapt to this major change in their lives. The children have an opportunity to discuss their feelings about the family as it has been and as they would like it to be. Their sense of involvement and control of their fate is considerably increased. Children's positive feelings for their parents are enhanced by seeing them cope well with conflict and crisis. In addition, parents experience less anxiety in this structured separation situation than in a comparable time negotiating for a final divorce. They thus are able to deal with their children's feelings more effectively. The separation counselor has an opportunity to help parents understand their children's reactions to the family crisis. He may then guide the parents so that they can encourage open exchange of feelings and concerns. Where necessary, the counselor may work directly with the children.

Viable relationships survive structured separation. Old patterns of thought, feeling, and behavior are broken. New patterns develop within each individual, between the couple, and even between parents and children. The couple's new relationship, whether a "together-relationship" or a "separate-relationship," is clearly based on choice rather than the force of circumstance, fear, default, or inadequacy.

THE SEPARATION STRUCTURE

The separating couple is asked to make a three month commitment to explore themselves and the relationship. During this time both will see the counselor—optimally once a week. They are seen both individually and together. Sometimes one comes regularly and the other only as he or the therapist deems necessary.

During this time the couple is asked not to live in the same house, not to see a lawyer, and not to make any permanent financial, property, or child custody arrangements. Children remain in their own home with whichever parent is best able to care for them. Their lives are disrupted as little as possible. It is important that they maintain contact with such environmental supports as friends and school. As the couple communicate with each other while realistically assessing their needs, they resolve practical issues. Decisions are made out of the awareness of both partner's needs, not out of fear, guilt, or revenge.

Each partner agrees to be together only if, when, how, and as long as BOTH are comfortable. This "choice" rule applies also to parent-child contacts. Each is free to initiate contact; each is free to end contact when he wants to, for whatever reason. The couple may have sex together only if both want to.

At the point of making the commitment to the separation structure, the couple is encouraged to express feelings about outside affairs. Freedom to explore other relationships is encouraged on the theory that such exploration maximizes choice. If the couple decides to come together again, each knows it is because he is desired over and above others. In addition, a variety of social, emotional and sexual encounters gives each a more realistic view of himself interacting with others. These contacts serve to eliminate "If it weren't for you" games. They also cut through the "I was too young and inexperienced," "Nobody else would want me," and "I had to get married" types of excuse for discontented clinging.

During these three months, the couple learns to relate to each other in terms of needs, feelings, qualities of being, defenses and games. The process of seeing each other only by choice requires that each examine himself and the other often to decide whether or not to be together and when and how to reject the other. In this process of repeatedly accepting and rejecting, each has an extraordinary opportunity to learn to be honest with the other in communicating love, appreciation, and need as well as hurt, fear, and anger. Each may thus learn to take responsibility for gratifying his own needs.

Honesty comes more easily during this structured separation because the couple now has little to lose. In choosing to face the ultimate loss, risks are taken which would not ordinarily be taken for fear of losing. The knowledge that one can survive financially and emotionally apart from the other and that there are alternative ways of gratifying needs breeds courage. Fears and grievances are expressed; catastrophic expectations of hurt, loss and guilt are seldom realized. The way is cleared for the more positive feelings. One client stated after a few weeks of structured separation:

> We are talking about everything, and I feel much more free and she more loved. I also no longer feel that divorce would be such a cataclysm that I couldn't do anything that might bring it up. It feels more like a real option now, than like a threat. However, we are both trying now to see that it isn't necessary. In any case it beats lying, and suicidal fantasies, and continual frustration; and on the other hand independence no longer seems so frightening. It feels like a choice between positives now, instead of between a negative and an unknown.

A new relationship EVOLVES out of a multitude of honest choices. This is a "let it happen" rather than a "make it happen" approach. If the couple establishes a new "together-relationship," it will be strongest if each one, being maximally himself and doing and being that which allows him most growth and satisfaction, also meets the other's needs and allows him to grow and be satisfied. Love develops when each satisfies the majority of the other's basic interpersonal needs without sacrificing his own need-satisfaction.

The following case illustrates the separation structure:

Mr. & Mrs. W. had children three and five years of age. Previous marriage counselors had been unsuccessful with this family. The W.'s had married because Mrs. W. was pregnant. She withdrew from school at age 17 and prematurely ended her adolescence. She resented her forced marriage, as well as her role as wife and mother. She wanted to return to school and to work. Mr. W. defined his manhood in terms of his ability to support his family. He held his wife to a high standard for housework, cooking, and child-care. He was demanding sexually, she was withholding.

The couple decided to divorce when Mr. W. discovered his wife's sexual involvement with a man six years her junior. Mr. W. then was uncomfortable about his decision and suggested they see another counselor. They subsequently agreed to delay their divorce for three months of separation counseling.

They decided to leave the children with Mr. W. in the family home. Their regular babysitter increased her time with them, thus providing consistent care while Mr. W. worked. The older child remained in school. Mrs. W. moved back to her parent's home, enrolled in night school and accepted a job. Mrs. W. did not ask for support money. She had managed the money for the family and knew there was not enough for two households. She visited the children three nights a week for their regular bedtime routine. They stayed with her at her parent's home every other weekend. The children were told the parents were having some problems being with each other now and were taking a vacation from each other for a while. Their difficulties were compared to difficulties the children had with their friends, where sometimes they didn't play together for a while.

Mrs. W.'s relationship with the young man ended a few weeks after her separation. She realized that she had involved herself with him more to express her resentment to her husband and to attempt to recapture her adolescence than because of the man's qualities. She dated heavily the first months of separation but found the men she now met were less interesting than her husband. She also found her sexual difficulties represented her own intrapsychic conflicts and were not specific to her husband.

Mr. W., formerly highly moralistic and socially inhibited, did not begin to date until the second six weeks of separation. The fact that other women found him attractive boosted his self-esteem. Simultaneously he began to define his adequacy in terms other than money and sex. Mrs. W. found him more attractive as he was desired by others. She enjoyed his new ease in relating.

At first, Mr. and Mrs. W. saw very little of one another. He left the house when she came over and cursorily left the children with her on the week-end. Gradually, he stayed home more often when she put the children to bed. They began to talk over their differences and discuss their present experiences and feelings. Mr. W. tended to be possessive and jealous; Mrs. W. gradually saw how she taunted him with subtle threats of abandonment. Mr. W. saw how he tried to hold his wife with ever-increasing, unsatisfiable demands. Mrs. W. became aware of her use of passive-aggressive, manipulative behavior which frustrated and angered him. She became more direct in her refusal to accede to his demands; more willing to risk openly defining and satisfying her needs. The couple explored new ways of solving problems through compromises. This couple also began to have fun together—a quality notably lacking in their marriage. They dated, danced, and played miniature golf once a week while still dating others.

During the three month separation period, Mr. W.'s homemaking duties led him to be more realistic in his housework and child-care standards. Mrs. W. enjoyed work, but found she did not enjoy school. With child-care voluntary, she found herself enjoying her children more and spending more time with them.

Sexual activities were resumed in the tenth week of separation. Intercourse was more satisfactory than it had been. Each was able to trust more and to be less controlling of self and other. With the diminution of frustration and anger, softness and warmth dominated their close time together. The sexual act became less important than the feeling between them.

The W.'s decided to reinstate their marriage after the twelfth week. Mrs. W. continued for a brief time in therapy to resolve her sexual conflicts.

SEPARATION COUNSELING

During the three month time period, the separation counselor needs to attend to three major areas. These are: (1) the individuals' response to the separation; (2) the individuals' basic quality of being; and (3) the together-relationship.

(1) RESPONSE TO SEPARATION: I have observed the following pattern among large numbers of separating people in singles groups and in clinical practice. People first experience a *shock reaction*. This is particularly obvious when the separation is sudden and unexpected. Most frequent expressions of this shock are denial and/or somatic disorder. Gastro-intestinal disturbances, headaches, changes in eating patterns and upper respiratory infections are common. These are best attended to by a physician. The therapist's role is to use the symptom as meaningful content and help the client openly experience the pain rather than deny, avoid, or internalize it.

The shock reaction is generally followed by an eight to 12 week *affective cycle*. The first phase of this cycle is characterized by a four to six week period of depression and withdrawal or by a similar period of euphoria and activity. During the following four to six weeks, those who have been depressed and withdrawn usually begin to feel more open and become more active. They seldom go as "high" as the group who were initially euphoric. Those who have at first been euphoric and active tend to withdraw and may become somewhat depressed. Again, the "low" tends to be less intense than that experienced by those initially depressed. This counterreaction gradually shifts and stabilizes at an intermediate affective and activity level. It is on this base that the person can best either grow as a single individual or begin to establish a new dependency relationship.

One of the separation counselor's important functions is to help each client accept himself and the other as each experiences the various phases of this affective cycle. This cycle represents a part of the normal response to loss. The period of withdrawal represents an unusual opportunity to introspect, to gain strength from one's own reserves, and to resist social pressure to "do something." The withdrawn period represents an opportunity to explore new directions that may be more meaningful than those followed before or during the marriage. This is a time when one may explore in fantasy plans to return to school, change employment, or even change careers. The excuse of "If it weren't for you and the marriage, I would have . . ." is, at least for the moment, not valid. This is a time to confront loneliness and to explore one's own resources. It is a time to become centered in oneself as a separate individual. The danger here is that couples will prematurely reunite in order to avoid pain. The therapist's assurance that this is a time-limited and normal depressive reaction and his encouragement to "go with it" helps clients use this period creatively.

The period of euphoria and activity may be a natural response to the temporary freedom from conflict and the need to make an immediate final decision. People often experience genuine pleasure with their new freedom. However, euphoria may, especially if extreme, represent an avoidance of depression and grief. The individual, the partner, and the children are more accepting of this activity if it is understood as a separation reaction. The separation counselor encourages the client to use his interactions at this time to learn about himself. As he engages in other relationships he is better able to understand himself, the marriage, and its failure. Repressed anger may pour out during this period of activity. This is particularly true for people who have played "good guy" in the marriage and have "done everything to keep the marriage together." This may also be a time in which the individual puts all of his energies into work. He may be particularly creative at this time, exploring and investing energy in new areas of competence.

Ambivalence is inherent to separation and is a prominent factor in the affective cycle. That the people stayed together at all indicates the existence of some positive value to the relationship. Some needs are still being gratified at the time of separation. The effectiveness and extent to which a couple gratified each other's needs in a positive way may be measured by the pain experienced on threat of loss. A great deal of negativity and anger also exists or the partners would not be separating. Most people find ambivalence difficult to sustain. It represents helplessness and loss of control. To cope with ambivalence requires the ability to tolerate nonstructure, frustration, conflict, inconsistency, and the simultaneous existence of opposites.

A very common way to cope with ambivalence is to focus on either the positive or negative ends, affective and attitudinal, of the spectrum. We find those who profess undying love and idealization of the relationship, despite a history of unhappiness and strife. More commonly, we find people who, after separating, hate and malign the other and who refuse to recognize the good that was in the relationship. Polarization may be extreme among people who have blocked from awareness one or more feeling states and who use emotions defensively. Thus, those who idealize often are afraid of their anger. Anger may be used to defend against tender feelings. It is often a defense against the pain of loss. Both anger and love may be used to avoid sadness, feelings of helplessness and hopelessness, or the need to face oneself. When therapist and client focus on the missing feelings, a more realistic emotional balance is attained.

Polarization of attitude, in addition to being a defense against ambivalence, may also be a symptom of decision making difficulty. When one cannot easily order data in terms of relative importance; or when one has depended on external events or people to determine one's life pattern, then there is a tendency to focus inappropriately on one aspect of a complex whole. The distorted view of the whole thus produced tends to make whatever decision one makes a foregone conclusion.

This 8 to 12 week affective cycle forms the basis for the three month time period found to be necessary for effective separation counseling. Both phases of this cycle represent adaptive reactions to the situation. Decisions made during this reactive period are often the result of such factors as relief that the pain of conflict is over, fear of the unknown, shame, and sense of failure. After the period of reaction to the past relationship and the separation situation, and after the individuals have used this time to fully assess themselves and their ways of being together, they can make decisions based on their present needs and value systems. Premature return to the marriage is avoided, as is premature and perhaps unnecessary separation or inappropriate rebound marriage.

The case of Mr. and Mrs. B. illustrates the importance of

working through the affective cycle. It also indicates the value of focusing on the individuals' quality of being.

Mrs. B., an aggressive social worker, came for help when her marriage was terminated by her husband, a shy engineer who had just finished school. He had discovered she had seduced his best friend. The couple was seen together once. Mr. B. refused to be involved in the structured separation process. Instead, he plunged into a relationship with an exotic dancer during the first week after rejecting his wife. Within a week after meeting, the dancer and her eight-year-old daughter moved in with him. They were later married but divorced after two years. Mr. B. had not been able to express anger directly before separation. Now, he expresses anger by withdrawing and withholding himself in a passive-aggressive manner.

Mrs. B. was advised to remain in therapy for at least three months so that she might be guided through the affective cycle. She began the cycle with a severe depression. She decided to "go with" the depression and take a sick-leave from work. When she thus "gave in," the colitis, which had begun when her husband rejected her, disappeared. The content of her therapy sessions were first dominated by self-castigation, anger directed at her husband, jealousy, and fear that she would never find another man. She now found the man she had seduced repulsive. She alternately idealized and denigrated her husband. She tried desperately to get him back. Her tears were of rage and helplessness. They also were manipulative. Gradually she began to accept her husband's adamant refusal to reinstate their relationship or even to explore the dynamics which led to her inappropriate behavior. With this acceptance of reality, she began to experience genuine sadness and to mourn the loss of her marriage and her husband. She had previously repressed tears of sadness, considering such tears a sign of weakness.

She returned to work after two weeks and functioned reasonably well. She avoided contact with men; had little contact with women. She became interested in returning to school and the possibility of a new profession. She had worked during the marriage to support her husband. It appeared that her need to control her husband was now being directed toward the control of her own life.

During the fifth week after beginning counseling, she entered into a sexual relationship that was, like her marriage, characterized by manipulations and hostility on her part. This relationship was explored in terms of her needs and intrapsychic conflicts and its similarity to her marriage. The relationship lasted about three weeks.

She began to shift toward the active part of the affective cycle during this relationship. First, she bought new clothes. Second, she moved to an apartment closer to the school which she planned to attend. This was in a neighborhood in which she had always wanted to live. She began phoning some old friends, going to office parties, and dating a few men. Her need to control and manipulate was a major focus of counseling. Her fear of emotional freedom was an important factor underlying this behavior.

During this part of the cycle, she began to find ways to talk to her husband directly, rather than manipulatively. She met his girlfriend and recognized the futility of changing his attitude toward her. They then were able to talk about their feelings for each other in the present and explored ways to end the marriage on good terms. He gave her emotional support while she cried and together they mourned the loss of their marriage. This interaction represented a rare moment in which Mrs. B. was able to trust another person to take care of her when she was feeling vulnerable. This inability to trust and to be comfortably dependent was a major reason for the failure of this marriage. Mrs. B. was advised to continue therapy beyond the three month period to resolve her dependency and control conflicts. She was not willing to do this. She followed through on her plan to return to school. She deepened her friendship with a man in her new apartment building and after a year, married him. That marriage has remained intact a year. In choosing this husband, she attended particularly to his ability to stand up to her controlling qualities.

(2) The Individual's Basic Quality of Being: How the indi-

vidual functions in general, aside from the specific separation situation, is an important area in separation counseling as it is in any therapeutic system. In separation counseling, emphasis is placed on the following factors: dependency and control needs and conflicts; the range of feelings available to the individual and how they are expressed; risk-taking behavior; ways of coping with loss; reactions to freedom; and value systems. Focus here in this area is more on individual growth and development than on the relationship.

Dependency and control patterns and conflicts become quite clear when the person on whom one has depended and controlled—or has been controlled by—is gone. These patterns become increasingly apparent in the new tasks for which each partner is now responsible, the way in which each accepts responsibility for himself, and what each seeks in others to supplement or complement his own perceived inadequacies.

During these three months the counselor helps the individuals to perceive and accept dependency and control needs and to find growth-promoting ways to satisfy them. The value of an equal and interdependent relationship is stressed. Manipulative maneuvers to insure security and control are discouraged; honest communication of needs and the willingness to gratify needs is encouraged.

An inability to experience and express the full range of *feelings* may have been an important factor contributing to the marital crisis. Emotional limitations will affect subsequent relationships. The counselor may take advantage of this time of stress to help open long closed emotional channels. Separation involves the arousal of a complex set of emotions. Some positive feeling is there, whether it be love, the memory of love, liking, or need. Sadness or grief is a natural concomitant of loss. Anger is always present as a response to the hurt and frustration of basic needs that bring people to the point of separation. Anger is a common response to the problems that accompany adapting to new ways of living. Fear almost always accompanies risk, and risk is an essential ingredient of change. People often experience some sense of helplessness and hopelessness. Many individuals find separation especially difficult because they remain hopeful when such hope is not warranted. Feelings of guilt and shame are also generally present.

The effective separation counselor is aware of "missing" emotions. He helps individuals (1) perceive their lack, (2) understanding how other feelings or thoughts are inappropriately substituted, and (3) develop an awareness of, and willingness to, in some way deal with those feelings heretofore repressed. Often such repression is accomplished by creating a fantasy image of oneself, the other, or the relationship. Such "defensive fantasies" do help the individual avoid certain feelings; they also prevent effective problem solving. Thus, in separation counseling, fantasy is replaced by the awareness of the reality of the situation. With this reality as a base, most problems and differences are easily resolved and the choice of leaving or maintaining the relationship is more easily made.

Risk-taking is inherent in the process of change that accompanies separation. The more risks one takes, the more opportunity for growth. This is a time for choice, change, and freedom. This is a time to "do your thing" honestly and openly; to "do nothing" during the depressed/withdrawn time; to engage the world in new ways during expansive times. This is a time when one can intensely experience every facet of existence.

Separation involves *role change*. Individuals change from marriage roles to single roles, perhaps from housewife to worker, from full-time parent to part-time parent, from accepted partner to rejected partner. A newly separated person must cope with the loss of old roles and "trained" reciprocal role-players. They must meet new role expectations and behavior.

Sometimes people who separate change their lives so extensively that they establish new roles and new role patterns. Or, they may maintain their former role patterns but find new people or situations to play the reciprocal role (i.e. a "helper" needs someone to "help"; a dependent person needs someone to depend on). In any event they must experience some disequilibrium while these patterns are in flux. The extent of distress experienced in making these role changes depends on the kinds of risk each takes and how gracefully and appropriately transitions are made.

Risk and change automatically involve *loss*. Each loss needs to be recognized as such and some consideration made of the meaning to the individual of the pattern and relationships lost, of his feelings about the loss, and how he goes about replacing the loss. Losses need to be mourned and thus made "finished business" (Tobin, 1971). The process by which one deals with loss is fully as important as establishing new behaviors, attitudes, roles, feelings or relationships to replace the old. (See Chapter IV, pg. 56.) How change is accomplished is as important as what change is made. Equally important is an awareness of reluctance to change and to risk. If one does not want to risk the unknown, he can gain much by learning to accept that to which he clings.

Separation makes new *freedom* suddenly available. Freedom can be frightening. Fear of freedom and its accompanying responsibility is found especially among individuals who need an external object for support, projection or control. Many couples separate in the belief that the other is restricting his freedom to experience life fully. Others cling to a relationship to avoid this freedom. Assessment of each individual's ability to use freedom at this time is helpful in alleviating conflict, clarifying dependency and control patterns, and the limitations each individual places on himself.

Value systems change over a period of years, but the changes are often not defined. Thus, for example, a couple may begin marriage with home and children agreed upon as a primary value. One partner may change and begin to place career or money above his family. Values placed on openness vs. secrecy, flexibility vs. rigidity, monogamy vs. sexual freedom, permissive vs. authoritarian child rearing often change for one and not the other. Or, it may be that before marriage, the couple did not believe that differences in these value dimensions were important. Making the individuals' values explicit helps both understand the basis for some conflicts. It also helps individuals make decisions, take risks, and clarify life goals.

Mr. and Mrs. A. agreed to separation counseling after a stormy 17 year sado-masochistic marriage. Mrs. A., a depressed, dependent, inadequate woman clung desperately to her alcoholic husband. Mr. A. felt trapped and angry. He was uncomfortable with his children. He found them intrusive and unsatisfying. He found his 11-year-old daughter sexually attractive; his 13-year-old son too much like his wife. Yet he feared divorce would damage the children more than his continued presence in the home. He did not believe his wife could cope with the children alone.

Mr. A.'s work led to his transfer to a city two hours from their home after a year of marriage counseling in which neither could leave the other. They decided to take this opportunity to try structured separation. Both continued to be seen weekly. The children were seen once.

The father visited the children sporadically; they visited him twice. He found the limited, structured time with them more comfortable than the unstructured time at home. He became more giving to them of material goods, less hostile, and in general a better masculine model. They grew less fearful and more accepting of him. With his change, they began to wish for his return home and to feel guilty for their parents' separation. The children's guilt was dispelled as the counselor and the parents helped them see the marriage more realistically.

Mrs. A.'s depression began to lift after separation. She became more openly angry with her husband as she felt less frightened by his physical presence. She worked through her fears and anger with the counselor so her negative feelings did not interfere with the children's more positive attitudes toward their father. Mrs. A. gradually took more effective control over the children and also became more giving of her time and attention to them. She transfered some of her dependency needs to them, some to women friends, some to the therapist.

It gradually became clear that she was better able to function when she was in control of her life. She became frightened and negativistic as soon as an adult made demands on her. Her children's demands were not so threatening. It also became clear that she was not so inadequate as she appeared to be.

Mrs. A. deepened her relationships with women friends. She dated a few times, but was too frightened of men to feel comfortable. She began to drink and frequent bars. This behavior was dealt with in therapy in terms of the needs her husband's alcoholism had gratified. In part, his nightly visit to the bar kept him away from home and allowed her to be alone. Yet, he earned enough money to support her and the marital status protected her. She used the marriage to maintain her position as a child with a harsh father. She had clung to it to avoid the problems of adulthood. Separation meant she had to risk being responsible for her own decisions.

Mr. A. had used his bar activities to avoid being at home. With separation and his own apartment, his drinking decreased. He enjoyed time alone after work and drank only on weekends. He was not depressed after separation, but he was relatively withdrawn and quiet. His pre-separation affective level had been dominated by anger; he now experienced more warmth and softness. In the second month of separation, he became involved with his secretary. She was a strong woman who enjoyed drinking and was not cowed by his authoritarian manner. Her strength allowed him to gratify his dependency needs. His self-esteem rose as he found his values and his way of being acceptable to her.

The couple's early contacts with each other were relatively long. They went out with friends who had not known of their separation. When alone, they were at odds with each other. Mr. A. continued to make sexual advances to which Mrs. A. reluctantly acceded. After the first month they saw each other only when he came for the children. Mrs. A. was now capable of openly rejecting him when she was uncomfortable in his presence. Mr. A. became less demanding. His self-worth became increasingly defined in terms of his own strength in equal interpersonal relationships, rather than in terms of his ability to dominate his family. They became less and less interested in each other as the three months came to an end.

This couple decided not to reinstate their marriage. A property settlement was made which insured the children's stay in the family home and psychotherapy for both children and mother. Alimony was arranged to be paid on a decreasing scale over a ten year period. This was intended to allow Mrs. A. to gain her strength, learn work-skills, and encourage self-sufficiency. This settlement was deemed advisable to discourage her use of helplessness to control others.

(3) THE TOGETHER RELATIONSHIP: The separation counselor attends both to the way the couple interacts during joint sessions and to the number and the quality of contacts outside of the counselor's office. The counselor works with them as he would in any joint therapy situation. In addition, he remains aware of the separation process and the way in which each is coping with it. He shares his awareness with the couple so that they may understand and work with separation-related behaviors in proper context. The time-commitment structure gives the counselor as well

as the couple the opportunity to work through situations which otherwise would very likely precipitate divorce (i.e., being open about sexual relationships with others). In the course of the three months, some couples, like Mr. and Mrs. W., continue to communicate, work through their differences, and learn more satisfactory patterns of mutual need gratification. By the end of the time, they choose to be together more often than they choose to be apart. They have proportionately more positive than negative interactions. These couples make a new together-relationship. Other couples spend enough time together to explore their relationship and to understand each other, and yet their time together leaves them unfulfilled. They tend to choose to be apart more often than they are together. At the end of the three month period they generally agree to finalize their separation. Some couples continue to be together more often than they are apart, but important conflicts remain unresolved. These couples may make a commitment to another period of structured separation; or they may structure a time-limited trial together-relationship. In the latter case, they are asked to make their own contract setting forth what each expects of the other and what each is willing to give to the other. Counseling continues until the couple are comfortable with a decision to come together or to part.

In a one-year follow-up of 18 couples who completed structured separation with counseling 6 reinstated their marriage and were satisfied with the new relationship, 12 divorced. Of these twelve, only one couple needed legal help in making a property settlement. All but one of the couples have maintained good feelings toward each other, and all feel they have made the right choice. One extremely dependent, border-line psychotic man experienced some disorganization of function for several months after finalizing the separation. The other 23 separating individuals had gained equilibrium as single people by the end of the time they agreed to finalize their separation.

SUMMARY

Structured separation with counseling offers couples in conflict a method by which they can use the separation crisis to maximize growth. Couples commit themselves to a three month period during which they agree to certain basic guidelines: to live apart; not to make any binding legal, financial, or child-custody arrangements; to be together only by *choice*. Prime importance is placed on values of choice, risk, and honesty.

By focusing on both individuals' reaction to separation, their personality structures, and their evolving together-relationship, a counselor's interventions help each partner through the various phases of the separation process.

At the end of the three month period, people generally have a firm understanding of themselves and their relationship. The decision whether to finalize the separation or reinstitute the together-relationship tends to evolve out of the time and counseling structure.

REFERENCES

Parad, J.: *Crisis Intervention: Selected Readings.* New York, Family Services Association of America, 1965.

Tobin, S.: Saying goodbye in Gestalt therapy. *Psychotherapy,* 8:150-155, 1971.

Toomim, M. K.: Structured separation with counseling: A therapeutic approach for couples in conflict. *Fam Process,* 11:299-310, 1972.

Chapter X

ALTERNATIVES TO DIVORCE AND THEIR IMPLICATIONS

GORDON A. HARSHMAN

- CONTINUATION OF THE STATUS QUO
- TRIAL SEPARATION
- RENEGOTIATION WITH ACCOMMODATION
- WORKING THROUGH TO CONSTRUCTIVE INTEGRATION
- ACTIVITIES

SEVERAL ALTERNATIVES ARE OPEN to the couple deciding on divorce. "To divorce or not to divorce" may be the only alternative being considered. Yet, there is more than one alternative to divorce and each has implications of great importance. These implications have relevance to each partner far beyond the decision of whether or not to divorce.

Lasting attitudes about one's basic nature and worth are at stake. There is a deeply rooted psychological need underlying the often heard statement, "I want to explore every possibility before giving up on our marriage." To give up too easily or quickly may lead to disturbing aftereffects. An identical decision arrived at through a carefully conducted, painstaking self-exploration may represent a significant turning point toward personal fulfillment. A similar level of self-exploration on the part of both marriage partners often results in a relationship best characterized as constructively integrated. Other alternatives to divorce include a continuation of the status quo, separation and renegotiation with accommodation. Each of these holds unique

167

significance for the marriage partner. Which is chosen depends upon the specific aspects of the situation, including the degree of understanding of the alternatives open and their implications.

CONTINUATION OF THE STATUS QUO

A decision to "try one more time" may have widely divergent results. Often the decision is made without serious analysis of the deeper issues, as may occur during an emotional reaction against divorce. The couple then often returns to essentially the same interaction pattern which had developed prior to the traumatic episode. Such a decision, if made without additional insight, has little chance of leading to a more satisfactory relationship. Some couples seem to go through cycles of frustration leading to blow-up or withdrawal, reaction with reconciliation, sometimes briefly satisfying involvement, then back to gradually building frustrations, etc.

In more fortunate circumstances some maturing experience on the part of one or both partners may enable a breakthrough toward a more satisfying relationship. Often, the "frustration cycle" is repeated until the couple separates in despair. Or, as with the couple who rarely constructively communicate openly, even in anger, a gradual withdrawal occurs.

The "status quo marriage" can usually be easily identified by a general atmosphere of unhappiness with bitterness or a sense of resignation. Although the couple remains together physically there is little or no meaningful communication or companionship.

Lacking basic skills of constructive communication and problem solving, attempts to improve the relationship flounder painfully and may be abandoned in despair. In essence, a *non*communication pattern is maintained and often exaggerated over the years. Open, honest and direct expressions of emotion are usually avoided, frequently in the misguided belief that such expressions will be misunderstood or result in destructive conflict.

Any personal fulfillment is usually achieved in spite of the marriage relationship, not within it. Such basic human needs as acceptance, personal growth, creative expression and self-actualization, if not stifled are met independently through work or individual activity and relationships, usually outside the home. A separateness, developed at first in self-protection, becomes the way of life, accepted if not welcomed. The "form" of marriage is preserved, without the spirit or functions basic to individual and mutual satisfaction and fulfillment.

In short, the implications of continuing an unhappy "status quo marriage" include avoidance of learning and practicing more effective communication skills, avoidance of direct open expression of feelings and the perpetuation of destructive cycles of conflict and/or withdrawal, often resulting in severely limited self-growth or mutual fulfillment.

Even a tacit, unspoken "decision" to avoid attempts to develop a more positive relationship postpones any real chance for achieving the deeper joys of the more open and constructive marriage encounter. Perhaps the only state more destructive of the human spirit than open hostile conflict is a state of deepening psychological withdrawal, a turning inward in resentment, bitterness or apathy. It is indeed regrettable that in the minds of so many "status quo" marriage partners, the openness and directness of potentially constructive and enhancing marriage encounter skills is confused with the destructive, tearing hostility which too often characterizes unskilled attempts to communicate. Determined to prevent destructive outbursts, one or both partners fail to realize the often disastrous nature of the decision to "control my emotions." If to "control emotions" is to "prevent expression of emotions" the opposite of working toward improved communication is usually achieved. Only by special effort can the process of repression be reversed. Yet such reversal must occur, at least to some degree, if the individual is to really gain "control of emotions" in the sense of 1) acknowledging their existence, 2) "owning" them, and 3) constructively and appropriately "expressing" them. And only through such positive and direct expression can the "self" truly be accepted.

The deeper implication of the "status quo" marriage, then, is the continued subjugation of the inner "self" of one or both partners, usually both. Even the dominant member of a dominant-submissive pair may be robbing himself or herself and partner of encounters which could add rich perspective. The other side of the coin pictures the submissive member cheating himself or herself and partner by withholding honest, growth-producing expressions of self.

Couples weighing the comparative advantages and disadvantages of "staying together" or divorcing often overlook these deeper considerations. A person can just as easily avoid discovering "self" by perpetuating a "status quo marriage" as through divorce. Divorce, if decided upon following deep self-exploration and careful analysis of interest patterns, values and basic personality characteristics of self and partner, may be a logical and growth-producing decision. It rarely is if decided upon in haste, without such self-exploration. The same personal characteristics and present communication inadequacies if not confronted, understood, and dealt with, will most often prevent the development of more satisfying relationships in the future. Either a person learns to "communicate" more effectively or he/she settles for proportionately limited interpersonal rewards.

Several suggestions for self-directed activities designed to increase self understanding and to improve the communication process are outlined at the end of this chapter. Experienced marriage counselors can suggest other such activities suited to the individual or couple. Keep in mind the fact, however, that serious use of such activities and/or the marriage counselor's help, will alter the "status quo"!

TRIAL SEPARATION

The couple seriously considering divorce may benefit from a temporary alternative, the trial separation. Such benefits, sadly, are too often myths conjured up through wishful thinking. However, if done with serious commitment on the part of each partner, and with specifically determined objectives, the trial separation can add a touch of reality perhaps unattainable otherwise. The words "serious commitment" hold the key.

Trial separation will mean something different to each couple. Details of such considerations as the following will differ, but are usually important in the process of setting up the experiment: which partner moves to the new location; how much physical distance will separate the two; whether or not "visiting" during the time of the separation will occur; the number of days, weeks or months of the separation; the kinds of objectives for which the separation is being conducted; and selection of acceptable ways of evaluating the degree to which each objective is achieved.

To assure optimal opportunity for success, the terms or details of the trial separation should be carefully worked out, understood by each partner, and accepted by each partner. If not, the trial separation may become just another step toward divorce. When terms are carefully and seriously worked out, this process itself may bring a new perspective into the relationship, and move the couple significantly toward a sound basis for the ultimate decision regarding divorce.

A significant implication of the seriously negotiated trial separation is that both partners are attempting to gain new understanding of self and their relationship. Neither partner has closed the door to renegotiation or working through their problems. Both have evidenced willingness to communicate during the negotiation stage of establishing terms for the separation. Both are committed to working toward achieving their mutually defined objectives, including periodic evaluation sessions.

Another implication of this alternative to divorce is that, somehow, one or both partners feel a need for more "space" or freedom during this time of critical evaluation. Where this becomes apparent it may be very helpful to analyze the closely related issues of "dependence-independence" and "need for territory." A counselor's help is usually needed for this rather complex procedure. A basic human need is to have both psychological and physical space. The basic need for privacy is often unrecognized, or discounted. Both a place and time for "aloneness" often seems vital to the process of personal renewal. In the case of the overly dependent person, there are often vague feelings of "I have no life of my own, no space of my own, no time of my own." The trial separation may provide a time for identifying such unmet needs and for developing plans to bring about needed changes, including the building in of "alone time" and more clearly identified territorial rights or space for personal belongings and activity.

A trial separation may also serve to exaggerate feelings of loss and awareness of the realities which would attend divorce. Especially in the case of longer term marriages, even a few days of total separation, with no communication of any kind, may be a great aid in clarifying the importance of the relationship. The new perspective gained may suggest a different order of personal priorities than previously acknowledged. Such insight may serve to unite a couple or at least provide a more concrete basis for divorce. Discovering how it feels to "wash my own socks" or "service my own car," etc., at times brings renewed appreciation for the spouse's role. Another reality quickly realized is the financial cost of maintaining separate quarters, only a part of the costs involved in divorce.

On the other hand, the perspective gained may be in the direction of realizing that few or no valid grounds for staying together really exist. One or both partners may decide there is no hope of developing a satisfactory level of common interests, mutual values and life goals; or that personality or life style conflicts are too deeply rooted to hope for achievement of even the minimal degree of change needed for a more compatible life together. Such awareness not only provides a more acceptable basis for deciding on divorce, but may add new insight in the establishment of future relationships.

RENEGOTIATION WITH ACCOMMODATION

The trial separation is at best a temporary situation. Under favorable conditions it will terminate in an acceptable reconciliation or in a decision for divorce based upon thorough self-exploration and objective analysis of the relationship. The nature of the relationship at the time of reconciliation, whether or not a trial separation is involved, may be categorized as one of the three basic alternatives to divorce: "continuation of the status quo," "renegotiation with accommodation," or "working through with constructive integration." The essential distinctions among these rather arbitrarily defined categories are 1) the level of effectiveness of communication, 2) the level of understanding on the part of each partner of his/her own and partner's life style —including values, needs, activity interests, and basic personality characteristics—and 3) the degree of acceptance of the various aspects of each other's life style.

The process of renegotiation with accommodation is nearly self-explanatory. The marriage relationship is analyzed and at least some points of conflict are resolved, resulting in an accommodation temporarily acceptable to both partners. The status quo has been significantly changed for the better. A communication process has been utilized which holds promise for periodic —or better yet, on-going—negotiation with progress toward fuller working through of temporarily tabled issues, with the further possibility of achieving the approach to problem solving characterized as constructive integration.

Negotiated accommodation, at least to some degree, reduces destructive conflict and results in an atmosphere more conducive of personal growth and satisfaction than is possible under the conditions of the "status quo" marriage. At the same time, it may be viewed as a desirable step in the lifelong process of constructive integration.

Several significant implications of this alternative to divorce can be identified. There is at least minimal self-exploration on the part of one or both partners. There is at least a minimal level of effective communication, with improved understanding of each other in a critical area of concern. A decision has been made that it is better, at least temporarily, to stay together than to divorce. There usually has been a successful effort to identify common interests, common needs, common values. Areas of disagreement or dissatisfaction have been identified and discussed. There has been at least a temporary accommodation or acceptance of perceived differences in needs, values, and behaviors. A basis for future negotiations has been established. There most likely remains much room for self-exploration and for improving communication skills, including skills in conflict resolution.

WORKING THROUGH TO CONSTRUCTIVE INTEGRATION

The fortunate couple who continue on the course outlined above are on their way to establishing the conditions for a more optimal human relationship. For this couple, the preliminary self and relationship analyses have indicated sufficient compatibility of basic life styles to warrant renegotiation of the marriage, with accommodation and at least temporary acceptance of unresolved issues. Some couples appear satisfied with such a degree of improvement in the relationship; others have discovered a life-long challenge leading beyond the more superficial and temporary "negotiation" stage to deeper levels of "working through" apparent differences to the point of constructive integration.

The couple moving in the direction of constructive integration have at least a partial understanding of processes which lead to increased self-awareness and personal fulfillment through mutually satisfying interaction. Processes which can open up unsuspected alternatives to divorce can also, if more fully understood and consistently applied, lead to the deeper and on-going satisfactions of self-actualization.

A key dimension, if not the core dimension, of self-actualization is an optimal level of interaction with other "selves." The optimal alternative to divorce demands incorporation of these constructive interaction components into the marriage relationship.

A behavior change of this magnitude, moving from a conflict state nearing divorce to an optimal human relationship, obviously is not going to happen quickly and without deep commitment on the part of both marriage partners. Insight and commitment to the hard and often painful work of unfreezing undesirable behavior patterns and the establishment of effective new patterns is a necessary beginning on the pathway to such a change. It is only that. The processes of constructive integration provide a framework or recipe for working through the backlog of unresolved issues which have temporarily been tabled; they also provide the necessary tools for resolving the many unforeseen issues of the future. This alternative to divorce demands a commitment to an on-going process of self-analysis and reevaluation of the communication process, and to the working through of perceived differences to the point of understanding and acceptance. There is no magic pill or process which once and for all guarantees harmony and happiness. Such a sentence is so trite as to be laughable, were it not for the sad fact that many couples act as if the opposite were true. Harmony and happiness in any long-term relationship are earned. And at times the price includes the temporary pain of confrontation, perhaps a necessary payment for a truly integrated and mutually fulfilling relationship. So, in addition to the prerequisites of insight and commitment, a third necessary condition is the understanding of and willingness to continuously apply the basic communication skills which are essential in the "working through" process. A corollary of this condition is the acceptance of the fact that application of the basic communication skills, especially in the process of conflict resolution, may be painful. Viewed as "growing pains," which is accurate when an issue is successfully worked through by means of effective communication procedures, confrontive interactions can become constructive building blocks, leading to new peaks of excitement and joy in an expanding relationship.

The term, "effective communication procedures," as given in any positive and meaningful relationship, in turn implies certain essential attitudes and skills on the part of the individual. Too often these attitudes and skills are taken for granted or assumed to be present when closer observation may indicate otherwise. Or invalid assumptions are made during human interactions about the various steps or processes involved. First of all there are the assumptions that the sender of a message, "A," 1) is really in tune with himself, therefore knows exactly what message he wishes to send, 2) actually sends exactly the message he intends, both through his words and nonverbally, and 3) is understood by the receiver of the message, "B." Secondly, on the part of "B," the receiver, there may be the assumptions that 1) "A" is sending the message he intends, even though he may not be, 2) "B" is hearing the message without distortion, which may or may not be true, and 3) that "A" knows exactly how his message was perceived by "B."

There are so many chances for error or distortion of meaning in both the "sending" and "receiving" processes of communication it is really to be wondered at when two people actually do communicate so effectively that both feel perfectly understood. A skill training activity such as the ones suggested at the end of this chapter can be most effective in helping a couple in the process of plugging communication gaps. Just being aware that "Mostly I neither send nor receive messages accurately" applies to everyone to some degree can be a significant step in itself. Such an awareness encourages frequent "checking out" to make sure a message is being sent or received as intended. Such a seemingly simple, kindergarten-like step may seem ridiculous or even offensive, but the fact cannot be overstressed that one of the major breakdowns or gaps in communication is failure to "check out." At the risk of seeming simple-minded or offensive, "Try it, you'll like it!" An exaggeration of the "checking out" step can be especially helpful in discussions of highly emotional issues. This is especially so because the process demands that "A" feel understood, whether or not "B" agrees with him, before "B" has a turn. Many arguments can be stopped or modified to the level of "discussion" by careful application of this one critical process.

Another implication in this alternative to divorce, and essential to the effective communication process, is that both partners are open to and skilled in receiving and giving feedback. The feedback process calls for an atmosphere of support and mutual respect and caring combined with open, direct honesty. Although these attributes may rarely exist in a pure form, there is little hope of really working through a major issue without some degree of each. Even an attitude of "Let's really try!" may ease the way to deeper levels of honest disclosure of feelings and help the couple hang in during the working through process.

The awareness that issues previously ignored or avoided can be brought into the focus of the "working through process" has beneficial and growth-producing effects beyond the solution of the immediate problem. Fuller understanding of self results in increasing self-acceptance and trust in both self and others, with increased risk-taking in a widening variety of situations. Fuller understanding of one's partner also leads to fuller trust in him or her. With increasing self-acceptance comes a decreasing of the fears of individual uniqueness, whether in self or partner. Parallel feelings of "I'm OK as is" and "You're OK as is" converge with an effect at times of ridding the self of a great weight. Such a breakthrough frees the individual to reassess his own and his partner's characteristics—assets and limitations, values, goals, interests—more objectively than ever before. A truly interdependent relationship becomes more and more an actuality, with each individual bringing strengths and needs to a relationship at once a union and strengthened by individuality and separateness. Along with increasing understanding and acceptance of the uniquenesses of each other comes a clearer understanding of areas of mutuality or compatibility of interests, values, behavior patterns and life goals, with a sense of well-being in relation to perceived future directions.

ACTIVITIES FOR IMPROVING SELF-UNDERSTANDING AND THE DECISION-MAKING PROCESS

Couples deciding about divorce need all available information and guidance. The following activities, designed to increase self-understanding and to improve the communication process, may be done in private or in a group setting. The couple may wish to consult a counselor, objective friend, or join a group with similar concerns, led by a competent facilitator. If engaged in with an attitude of commitment to make decisions based on the fullest possible information and real concern about effects on both partners, such activities can be most helpful.

1. When in doubt, consult a Counselor
2. "Plugging Communication Gaps" (The basic activity for improving the communication process)
   Objectives:
   1) To emphasize the key steps in effective verbal communication.
   2) To point out some common pitfalls or gaps in the communication process.

3) To provide a guide for conflict resolution.

Procedures:

1) "A" identifies a message he/she would like to send to "B."

2) "A" sends the message (as clearly, directly and concisely as possible).

3) "B" receives the message.

4) "B" checks out with "A" to make sure the intended message has been accurately received. This includes asking for clarification as needed and "playing back" to "A" the message that has been received.

5) "A" either accepts "B's" playback as accurate or corrects "B" until sure the intended message has indeed been accurately received.

6) "B" sends his response, if any, becoming the "sender," with "A" becoming "receiver," and steps 2-5 are repeated.

Caution:

1) "B" must convince "A" that "A's" message has been accurately received *before* sending his/her own message.

2) Be aware that the sender at best approximates sending the message actually intended. That, furthermore, the "intended" message may be fuzzy or only partly clear.

3) Be aware that the receiver, usually without knowing it, "screens" all incoming messages to fit his own needs and perceptions, thus the chance of receiving even a well-sent message exactly as intended is slight; distortion is especially apt to occur during emotional interactions.

4) Step 4 is critical and often omitted, especially during a heated argument; when included, arguments (or conflict) often become manageable and may be turned into constructive encounters.

5) The receiver may overlook the nonverbal messages which may be much different from the verbal; be sure to acknowledge such, without interpretation. Try to re-

spond to the *central* message, whether verbal or non-verbal, in the "playback" step.

Time needed:

No certain amount of time. It is suggested that couples practice the step-by-step procedure on a nonthreatening topic.

3. "I, You, We like. . . ."

Objective:

To identify mutual activity interests.

Procedures:

1) Each partner lists in three columns those activities enjoyed by self, by partner, and by both.

2) Partners share lists, discuss implications.

Time needed:

30-60 minutes.

4. "What Do I Gain, Lose by Staying With You?"

Objective:

Clarify basis for decision regarding divorce.

Procedure:

1) List on separate sheets "What I will gain" and "What I will lose" by staying with *(Partner's name).*

2) Partners share lists and discuss implications.

3) Revise lists and repeat step 2.

Time needed:

Probably several hours, in a situation free of interruption. (This activity can be modified for clarifying decision as to whether to do a trial separation.)

5. "Personal Log or Dairy"

Objective:

Deepen self-awareness and level of communication, especially during times of stress.

Procedures:

1) Keep personal log or diary of significant events, reactions, feelings, decisions.

2) Partners share selected items or in full at mutually selected times.

Time needed:
Varies; special need for privacy.

6. "Who Am I?" (Role Identification/Role Stripping)
   Objective:
   Increase understanding of self and partner in areas of basic values, interests.
   Procedures:
   1) Identify the things in life (roles, activities, etc.) which are most important to you, which make you what you are.
   2) List each one on a separate 3 x 5 card or slip of paper.
   3) Arrange in order from most to least important and number them accordingly.
   4) Share with partner, explaining the significant reasons for order of importance, etc.
   5) Partners arrive at equal number of items by having person with most items remove the least important ones.
   6) Taking turns, remove one item at a time, explaining to your partner the basis for your decision as to which to remove.
   7) Repeat this process until all items, or all but one have been stripped away.
   Time needed:
   Allow 45-60 minutes.

7. "Who Am I?" (Assets, Liabilities)
   Objective:
   To improve understanding and objectivity regarding real and perceived personality characteristics, abilities and limitations of self and partner.
   Procedures:
   1) Each partner privately lists what he/she perceives his/her assets (strengths) and liabilities (weaknesses) to be, using separate sheets or columns. Heading of page: "What I perceive my strengths/weaknesses to be."
   2) Do the same for partner, using heading, "What I perceive *(Partner's Name)*'s strengths/weaknesses to be."

3) Partners share lists. Caution: Avoid getting "stuck" by going entirely through both lists before stopping for discussion, except to check out meanings.

4) Variation: Partners may gain additional insight by adding columns headed "How I think *(Partner's Name)* sees my assets/liabilities" and "How *(Partner's Name)* think I see her/his assets/liabilities."

Time needed:

Allow at least an hour for steps 1-3. Extended discussions usually follow.

8. "Where Am I?" (Lifeline)

Objectives:

1) To identify the significant experiences in your life—those which have helped make you who you are.

2) To clarify current life style and feelings about it.

3) To provide a basis for personal goal setting, with increased sense of control in planning for the future.

Procedures:

1) Draw line lengthwise across middle of paper. Write word "Birth" at left end, present date near right end of line.

2) Place a plus sign (+) at top of paper on left side, a minus sign (−) at bottom to indicate whether experience was positive or negative.

3) Divide center line into time periods—Early Childhood (ages 1-10), Adolescence (11-20), Early Adulthood (21-30), Later Adulthood (31 ff). Leave room at the right for inclusion of current or recent experiences.

4) Select a minimum of two or three significant experiences for each time period. "Experiences" include significant relationship with others, school or career experiences or accomplishments, and personally fulfilling experiences or achievements such as hobbies, sports, etc., as well as "happenings" of a "one of a kind" nature.

5) Indicate where each falls on your lifeline by placing a mark and a word or two to identify the experience

in the appropriate position on your lifeline. Amount of distance above or below the lifeline indicates how positive or negative that particular experience was to you *at that time.*

6) Draw a "line of best fit" to indicate your over-all feeling about your life through the years from birth to present.

7) Observe how far above or below the center line your "lifeline" falls at various periods of time, and the kinds of experiences that account for negative or positive shifts.

8) Share your lifeline with your partner. You may wish to add events to your lifeline that come to mind as you share.

9) Identify the kinds of experiences which a) you wish could happen more often or b) you wish to avoid in the future.

Time needed:

1½ to 2 hours.

9. "Where Am I Going?" (Goal Setting)

Objectives:

1) To clarify values, interests, and desired future directions.

2) To define and establish short and long term goals.

3) To determine how to fulfill each goal.

Procedures:

1) First do activities #6 and #8 ("Role Identification/ Stripping" and "Lifeline")

2) Identify those roles or experiences you would most like to achieve or spend your time (life) doing in the future.

3) Make a new set of cards, one for each role or experience identified in step #2.

4) Number your items according to their relative importance or priority in your life.

5) Share your priorities with your partner, discussing their implications.

6) Setting goals: Select a high priority item and determine exactly what you would like to do about it in the future. Make a goal statement, i.e., "I want to be a better Father." (Repeat step 6-9 for other items.)

7) Identify specific objectives which spell out exactly what must be done to achieve your goal, i.e., "To become a better Father, I will 1) spend more time doing things with my son that are enjoyed by both of us, 2) let him know I understand his problems, 3) etc."

8) Develop an "action plan" for meeting each goal. Decide *what* to do, *how* to do it, under what circumstances, etc.

9) Determine ways and times for checking up on yourself as to progress being made. You may need to modify your goal or objectives, try a new approach or change your time table.

10) Share goals and action plans with partner, incorporating each other's suggestions where possible. Openly stated goals and plans add to sense of commitment.

Time needed:

Minimum of 2 hours.

10. "What I Like about You Is. . . ."

Objectives:

1) Identifying attractions to partner.

2) Stating positive feelings openly.

Procedures:

1) "A," "What do you like about me?"

2) "B," "What I like about you is. . . ."

3) "A," "You like. . . ." (Playback, checkout each statement)

   Caution: Avoid tendency to argue or play down positive feedback; it may help to keep a record.

4) Take turns doing steps 1-3 until each feels all significant "likes" have been stated and heard.

Time needed:

30-60 minutes.

11. "Surfacing Resentments"

Objective:

To work through the layers of hostility as a step in identifying, expressing and expanding feelings of tenderness and love.

Procedures:

1) "A" asks, "What do you resent about me?"
2) "B" responds, "I resent you when. . . ."
3) "A" checks out, to make sure the message is heard and
   understood.
4) Repeat steps 1-3, taking turns, until all resentments are
   surfaced and heard.

Time needed:

Varies, but allow minimum of 1-2 hours for activity and
discussion. Several sessions with breaks between may be
desirable.

12. "Role Reversal"

Objectives:

1) Gain understanding, empathy for partner's position,
   feelings.
2) Conflict resolution.

Procedures:

1) Select a point of controversy in which one or both
   partners is confused or cannot seem to understand the
   other's position or feelings.
2) Each partner assumes the role of the other. Attempt
   to say what the other has been saying, or what you
   imagine she/he would say, with the emotional expressions that fit. Try to "be" your partner.
3) After a few minutes stop and check out accuracy of
   the role portrayed.
4) Repeat the role reversal process as needed until each
   partner is satisfied that the other is at least fairly accurate in the portrayal.
5) Discuss implications of new insights.

Time needed:

Varies.

13. "Unlocking the Stereotype Cage"

Objective:

To distinguish which resentments toward partner may be due (at least in part) to unresolved resentments toward another important person (parent, sibling, other).

Procedures:

1) "A," "You remind me of (other person's name) when you. . . ." (Be very specific in describing which behaviors remind you of the other person)
2) "B" listens, checks out, plays back message.
3) When "A" is satisfied that "B" has the message, "B" has a turn.
4) Discussion might include:
   a) "What this means to me is . . . ,"
   b) "What I'd like to do about this is . . . ," and
   c) "What I wish you would do is. . . ."

Time needed:

Varies.

14. "Nonverbal Charade"

Objectives:

1) Clarify deeper feelings toward partner.
2) Get feelings into open, to provide basis for discussion.

Procedures:

1) Taking turns, act out deepest feelings toward partner, using no words.
2) Partner feeds back verbally when message is clear.
3) Several rounds may be desirable, as process often helps an individual work through one feeling to the point of allowing others to surface.

Caution:

1) Be sure the first partner feels understood before going to the second round.
2) Mutually determine in advance the necessary limitations on "acting out," especially if hostility is to be expressed. Beating a cushion, using a padded bat (bataca), etc., are excellent alternatives to broken heads. When in doubt, do this activity under the supervision of a counselor or other objective third party.

Time needed:

Allow at least an hour per round for first session. Later "charades" may take less time.

15. *References*

Additional activities may be suggested by your counselor. The following books are also excellent resources in the process of improving self-understanding and the basis for decisions about marriage and divorce:

Bach, George R., and Wyden, P.: *The Intimate Enemy: How to Fight Fair in Love and Marriage.* New York, W. Morrow & Co., 1968.

Gunther, B.: *Sense Relaxation: Below Your Mind.* New York, Macmillan, 1968.

Johnson, David W.: *Reaching out: Interpersonal Effectiveness and Self-Actualization.* Englewood Cliffs, New Jersey, Prentice Hall, 1972.

Otto, H. A.: *Group Methods to Actualize Human Potential: A Handbook.* Beverly Hills, The Holistic Press, 1970.

Otto, H. and Otto, Roberta: *Total Sex.* New York, Peter H. Wyden, Inc., 1972.

Pfeiffer, J. W. and Jones, J. E.: *Structured Experiences for Human Relations Training.* Iowa City: University Associates Press, 1970, 1971 (3 volumes).

Schutz, W.: *Joy: Expanding Human Awareness.* New York, Grove Press, Inc., 1967.

Stevens, J. O.: *Awareness: Exploring, Experimenting, Experiencing.* Lafayette, California, Real People Press, 1971.

Please comment on any of these questions which, from your experience, you have some feeling about. Use additional sheets where needed.

1. Social advantages, disadvantages of different types of housing?

2. Meaningfulness of religious institutions in meeting *social* needs?

3. Meaningfulness of living with roommate(s)?

4. Meaningfulness of individual psychotherapy or group therapy in enhancing adjustment? In what ways?

5. Meaningfulness of seeking further education as a means of enhancing social adjustment?

6. Meaningfulness of "singles" bars?

7. Meaningfulness of joining such groups as the Ski Club, Wine-Tasting Society, Art Museum, Sailing Club, Flying Club, etc.?

8. The importance of a work setting—is one setting worse or better than another in enhancing social adjustment?

9. Role of sex in dating patterns—what may a "newcomer" expect today?

10. Adjustment immediately following separation—what helps?

11. Special problems created by a long period of separation, prior to anticipated divorce? Advice?

12. Special problems created by being a woman, and advice to other women?

13. Special problems created by being a man, and advice to other men?

14. Special problems created by being of a certain age—e.g. under 20 or over 40, and advice to others?

15. Importance to social adjustment of having largely uncommitted leisure time, in contrast to not being "available"?

16. What may an individual expect when confronting the idea of being single, after having been accustomed to the social supports of marriage?

Chapter XI

ORGASMIC PROBLEMS: A COUNSELING DEMONSTRATION

ALEXANDER P. RUNCIMAN AND E. LEE DOYLE

THE MATERIAL PRESENTED is from the 1969 annual meeting of the American Association of Marriage and Family Counselors held in Dallas, Texas, November 7, 8, and 9, 1969. The following material is entitled "Orgasmic Problems—A Counseling Demonstration." Panelists include the following: Dr. Harold Lief, Professor of Psychiatry, Director of the Division of Family Study, Director of the Marriage Counselors of Philadelphia, Director of the Center for the Study of Sex Education in Medicine, all these directorships at the University of Pennsylvania.

The next panelist is Dr. Alex Runciman. Alex is from Southern California. He earned his Ph.D. in Sociology from the University of Southern California. He has spoken nationally to medical associations and various societies on the facts and the fallacies of sexual response. He is currently in private practice in Van Nuys, California.

The next panelist is Dr. Lee Doyle. Lee earned her Ph.D. in Family Life from Florida State University and presently is in Dallas in private practice, and teaching Marriage and Family at the Texas Woman's University. She has 12 years of university teaching and experience as a therapist at the Human Development Clinic and the Marriage Counseling Clinic at Tallahassee treating both children and adults with psychological problems. Runciman and Doyle were the first co-therapy team trained by Masters and Johnson and spent one year at the Reproductive Biology Research Foundation as Co-therapists and Research Associates. They are both members of this association.

The next two panelists are our experts in drama and the credits you see relate only to that talent, not to the talents that most

188

know them by. Dr. Laura Singer Magdoff is the wife of a film producer and has appeared in many TV shows including "For Women Only," "Youth Forum," "Council of Churches," and "Today's Woman." She is frequently heard speaking on sex education and the generation gap. She is Past President of the American Association of Marriage and Family Counselors.

We have equally good credits for the male member, Dr. Jim Peterson who is a member of the American Federation of Television and Radio Actors. He has produced many dramatic shows on his own including "For Better or for Worse," "Conflict in Marriage," "The House Party." He is also Past President of the American Association of Marriage and Family Counselors.

Dr. Lief will conduct an initial interview with the couple coming for counseling. The role playing couple are our own two A.D.M.F.C. members who gladly and kindly volunteered. Incidentally, Laura's role will be that of a nonorgasmic female. After the initial interview we will hear Dr. Runciman and Dr. Doyle who were the first co-therapy team with the Master and Johnson research foundation. They will give us an insight of how they would work with this couple using the background information that has been produced.

Dr. Lief: Mr. and Mrs. Peterson, will you be comfortable if I use your first names? What would you like to be called, Jim?

Jim: That's all right Doctor.

Laura: Laura.

Dr. Lief: Now while you are making yourselves comfortable, I wonder if you will give me. . . .

Jim: Doctor, I don't want to interrupt but I have a business meeting in half an hour, so let's get at it.

Dr. Lief: Okay.

Laura: Everything else is more important than I. Everything!

Jim: Well, damn doctors, this is the third one.

Dr. Lief: Tell me a little bit about your past experience.

Jim: It's her problem. Let her tell you.

Laura: What do you mean, it's my problem? All right. It's my problem. I wanted to come here because I don't think I can continue to live with Jim. I really don't.

Jim: She never has lived with me. That's the problem.

Laura: That isn't true.

Jim: What do you mean, that isn't true?

Laura: Well, you lie. You lie all of the time. You know damn well that I have lived with you. Weren't we together? You know what he means when he says lived with.

Dr. Lief: Tell me.

Laura: He means that we don't have sex. As much as he would like to have sex.

Jim: Huh! Much as I get it, once every month. Once every two months.

Dr. Lief: Just hold things a moment. We will get into this in a second. How many years have you been married?

Jim: Two. Two too many.

Laura: Not quite. Two too many but it's not quite two years.

Dr. Lief: Is this the first marriage for both of you?

Laura: Yes.

Dr. Lief: Any children?

Laura: No.

Dr. Lief: Now tell me about the problem as you see it. Oh, before we do that, how did you happen to come here?

Laura: My gynecologist suggested that we come to you and we thought it was a good idea. At least I thought it was a good idea. Jim doesn't think anything is a good idea, anything that I suggest.

Jim: The gynecologist said she should come.

Laura: What do you mean he said I should come? You know it's —oh well. Go ahead.

Dr. Lief: Apparently you are not very happy being here. Tell me about your feelings coming here.

Jim: Doctor I'm a very busy man. I have a meeting in half an hour. Let's get on with it.

Dr. Lief: That's all the time we have so we will have to make the best use of that time. What are your feelings about coming here?

Jim: I've tried every way for two years to make this girl happy. I work ten to twelve or fourteen hours a day to give her the things she demands, then she bitches, bitches, bitches and never gives me anything in return.

Dr. Lief: How do you feel about it?

Laura: How do I feel? I think he's crazy. He thinks he's giving me everything. You think you are giving me everything. What in the hell do you give me? Nice clothes, you think that's everything?

Jim: What you ask for. The house, the new car, the fur, and every one of them, give me, give me, give me, but you give me nothing back.

Laura: You know you like to give me things. You always tell me that you like for me to look nice.

Jim: I wanted you to look nice. Now I give a damn, really. I wish you would look nice in bed sometime.

Laura: If you gave me a chance, maybe I would look nice in bed but you are all over me all the time. You're all over me. I cannot lie there. I can't do anything, you just grab at me all the time.

Jim: Well, if we had a normal sex life I wouldn't be all over you. Once every six weeks.

Laura: Oh come on, you've always turned me off.

Jim: That is the truth. During the first of our marriage I caressed you, I loved you forty minutes, fifty minutes, an hour, it didn't do a damn bit of good and you know it.

Laura: Well you know that I told you I was slow. I told you that it was hard for me. You said that you would understand.

Jim: I understood for a year.

Laura: What do you mean, you understood for a year? You only tried that once or twice and then you did all those awful things to me.

Jim: What awful things?

Laura: The things I couldn't stand. You know what I mean.

Jim: You said let's experiment to try to help you.

Laura: Yes, but how you did it, how you did it. Do you know how rough you are? You hurt me all the time. I thought you loved me.

Jim: Love you! I had 56 girls before I was married.

Laura: Why didn't you marry them?

Jim: Well, I should have! Not one of those girls had problems and I treated them the same way.

Dr. Lief: What was it like before marriage?

Jim: It wasn't any good with her before marriage either but. . . .

Laura: You said it would be better afterwards.

Jim: I said we would try afterwards. Maybe if you were a little more secure it would work out. But it hasn't been any different. You've been this way ever since I knew you, before marriage and during the first year. You know it.

Laura: You don't give me a chance. You never did. You just grab at me and you leap at me and you are just there, all over me all of the time. I can't stand it.

Laura: Really when he tried, when he tried at the beginning, I felt better. I felt as though. . . .

Jim: Oh hell, she. . . .

Laura: As though, maybe, something would happen. A little bit more. But then he gets so impatient. . . .

Jim: She didn't feel a thing, Doctor. Let me tell you. . . .

Laura: Oh come on, how do you know what I felt?

Jim: You used to turn away from me after a half an hour.

Laura: Well because it got so, I felt bad, I felt bad.

Dr. Lief: What do you mean, Laura?

Laura: Well, because first of all, you know, I felt as though I should be doing something else. I didn't know what else I should be doing.

Dr. Lief: You blamed yourself?

Laura: Yes, well he was blaming me all the time, of course, I blamed myself.

Dr. Lief: And apparently you have been to other people for help over this. Was the gynecologist the first person you were able to talk to about this?

Laura: He was the first.

Dr. Lief: So this is the first time you have asked for professional help?

Laura: Yes.

Dr. Lief: What did the gynecologist tell you about your problem?

Laura: Well, he just thought that there was something that I wasn't seeing right or maybe that I wasn't responding as fully as I might be able to and so he suggested that maybe we come here, that maybe the two of us together could do something. He was very kind.

Dr. Lief: What do you expect of a marriage counselor? What are you looking for, Jim?

Jim: Well, I'm not expecting very much. Something is wrong with her. She can't respond. She never has. What do you think we should expect?

Dr. Lief: You've been angry with her since the day you were married? Or did that develop later?

Jim: Well, we fought a great deal before marriage.

Laura: We didn't fight all that much.

Jim: Oh hell! You wanted to live in Chicago. We couldn't live in Chicago. We fought about that. You wanted your mother and we couldn't have your mother, or I wouldn't have her. We fought before marriage.

Laura: Yes. . . .

Jim: And you kept saying "after marriage Jim, after marriage Jim." It's been hell.

Laura: I thought it would be different. I thought if we lived together and we got to know each other it would be different. But it isn't different, it's worse.

Dr. Lief: Were there ever tender moments? Were there times when you had fun together, when it was a delight to be with each other?

Laura: Oh, there are times when it is fun. I think.

Jim: Very few, Doctor, very few.

Dr. Lief: Apparently that was so even during your courtship?

Jim: Yes.

Laura: Well, why did you marry me then? You told me you loved me and you wanted me. Why did you marry me?

Jim: Well, I thought you could be normal.

Laura: Doctor, what does he mean when he says that I could be normal? What does that mean?

Dr. Lief: Laura, have you ever had a climax?

Laura: No.

Dr. Lief: Not with Jim? Never with self-stimulation?

Laura: No. It was nice but I have never had a climax.

Dr. Lief: You must have engaged in petting when you were in college?

Laura: Yes, I did.

Dr. Lief: And during all those experiences you never had a climax?

Laura: Sometimes it was very close.

Dr. Lief: You felt that you could?

Laura: I just felt that with a little more patience, or a little more time, a little more something but it just never happened.

Dr. Lief: Jim, how do you feel about the situation? Do you see the possibility of your doing anything to help Laura to achieve this?

Jim: Well I told you I tried during the first year. I was patient, I was kind, I gave her everything.

Laura: Oh, you were not. Oh come on, Jim, that's a lie.

Jim: I made love to her by the hour. . .

Laura: That's an absolute lie. How can you lie like that? You know what you did. You just grabbed at me.

Jim: Not in the beginning I didn't.

Laura: Just for a little while you didn't, a little while, maybe the first month.

Jim: The first year.

Laura: Oh come on, it wasn't a whole year.

Jim: Well, I got tired. There was no response.

Laura: I don't know what kind of response you want.

Jim: I want you to be normal, to like me, to like to be caressed and to be loved.

Laura: I like to be caressed but the way you caress me, I don't like it.

Jim: Oh hell, when I come home, Doctor, at night and I don't put my arms around her—huh!

Laura: That's because what happens—what happened this morning, remember?

Jim: What happened this morning? Nothing has happened for months.

Laura: Oh come on, it happens.

Dr. Lief: What is it? What did happen?

Laura: Well, when he, he grabbed at me when I am just about to get up in the morning and that's when he gets so passionate. He can't keep his hands off me and I don't even want it then. I'm not interested then.

Jim: Doctor, what do you expect? No sex for six weeks.

Dr. Lief: And are there times when she's more receptive, Jim?

Jim: She's never receptive. . . .

Laura: Oh come on, Jim. You know what happens when we go out sometimes and we dance and we come home and we've had a good time.

Jim: Yeah, I put my arms around you and after a while you say "goodnight."

Laura: You know why. How do you put your arms around me? You're not telling—you're not leveling. You really aren't. You're not telling the truth.

Jim: What's the truth?

Laura: The truth is the way you grab at me. If you were more tender with me it would be different but you're not tender. You grab at me and if I don't respond right away you just get mad and I feel like I don't want to have anything to do with you.

Dr. Lief: What about the other areas in your marriage?

Jim: Well we are doing all right. I'm the head of a company and we have a nice house and I would like to have some children there. She doesn't want any children. She's afraid of children.

Dr. Lief: How about that?

Laura: I am afraid. I think sometime I might have some children but, well, my mother said she had a terrible time when I was born.

Jim: Tell him what else your mother said.

Laura: I got scared.

Jim: Tell him what else she said.

Laura: I got scared when she said it hurt.

Jim: Tell him what else she said about sex. Tell him.

Laura: I don't have to tell him anything I don't want to tell him.

Dr. Lief: You've heard a lot of stories about the difficulties women have giving birth.

Laura: Yes. I'm scared. I don't want to go through all of that.

Dr. Lief: Have you talked to your gynecologist about that?

Laura: That's why he sent me to you.

Dr. Lief: What kind of contraceptive measures do you use?

Laura: I use a diaphragm.

Dr. Lief: Do you have any difficulties with it?

Laura: Well, at the beginning there was. I didn't like it. Kind of messy. But now I'm kind of use to it.

Jim: The gynecologist told her every night she should insert the thing.

Laura: I can't do it every night. I don't feel like doing it every night.

Jim: You don't feel like doing it any night.

Laura: That's not true.

Jim: Well, I wish you would wear a sign or something.

Laura: If you were smart you would see the signs. I wouldn't have to broadcast them.

Jim: When I do feel tender and I want to make an. . . .

Laura: When is that?

Jim: Let me talk, will you?

Laura: When do you feel tender, Jim?

Jim: Well, I feel tender quite often. You know it. And I show it and. . . .

Laura: I don't call that being especially tender. . . .

Jim: And you just push me away. . .

Laura: That's just being sexy, that's not being tender.

Jim: Okay, I don't get close enough to you to be rough to you.

Laura: You don't get close. You grab at me.

Jim: Yeah, but I never reach you.

Laura: Oh, come on.

Dr. Lief: Do you ever see him be tender?

Laura: I saw him tender at the beginning. Then he was tender and then I thought it was good and that we would have a chance at something. . . .

Jim: Good hell!!!

Laura: And then he turned off.

Jim: Who turned off?

Laura: Well. . . .

Jim: Who turned off? Who turned off?

Laura: Well, I turned off because you got so rough. You think you are giving me pleasure and you are hurting me and I tell you that you are hurting me and you say "oh there you go again."

Jim: Anything hurts you.

Laura: It isn't true but you do hurt me.

Jim: Doctor, about two weeks ago I came home and said I'm going to try again. You know how it is. You say, "Oh well, I'm going to try again." I came in and I had roses. I gave them to her and I said, "I love you" and I tried to put my arms around her and she backed off. How in the hell can I be tender with a woman like that?

Laura: Just because you brought me roses, you expect me to be tender. What happened that morning? What happened before you left?

Jim: You turned me off again that morning.

Laura: You grabbed at me again.

Jim: I wouldn't grab at you if I ever had any response. Any normal man. . . .

Laura: Here we go again, oh wow!

Dr. Lief: If you are so afraid of getting pregnant and having children, does this make any sense to you that this might be important in the way you respond sexually?

Laura: I hadn't thought about it. I hadn't thought that but it does make sense. Oh, but I wear a diaphragm.

Jim: Huh!

Dr. Lief: But how sure are you of its protection?

Laura: I guess I'm pretty sure.

Dr. Lief: You are pretty sure?

Laura: I haven't really thought about it.

Dr. Lief: Well since the pill is a lot safer, why haven't you thought of taking the pill?

Laura: I've heard an awful lot about the pill. All kinds of things happen to you, thrombosis and stuff.

Dr. Lief: You're scared then.

Laura: I'm scared of them.

Jim: Doctor, she's scared of everything. Tell them about your driving on the freeway.

Laura: What has that got to do with sex?

Jim: It's got a lot to do with it.

Dr. Lief: What Jim?

Jim: She's just frightened. She can't drive on the freeway. . . .

Laura: All those cars rushing at me. I do get scared. But what has that got to do with sex?

Jim: You're afraid of the diaphragm. You're afraid of having a child. You're afraid of the freeway. You're. . . .

Laura: I'm not afraid of the diaphragm. I'm afraid of the pill. You've got it wrong.

Jim: You're afraid of your mother.

Dr. Lief: You are afraid of the pill but you are not quite certain of the diaphragm.

Laura: I thought I felt pretty good about the diaphragm. I really didn't know that I didn't, you know, that I had some bad feelings about it.

Jim: She never uses it.

Laura: Honestly Jim. You say never, all. . . .

Jim: The gynecologist said you should use it every night and then if things happen you wouldn't have to get up. It's a hell of a way to have sex.

Dr. Lief: Laura, let me ask you a few questions about your childhood. What—You've already spoken about your mother giving you some ideas about the pain of childbirth. What was the general atmosphere in regard to sex?

Laura: Well, I knew that you have sex in marriage and I knew that I was expected to have sex in marriage and sometimes I thought it would be fun and sometimes I thought that it would not be such a good idea. I thought that there would be some other kinds of things that would happen but I was sure that when I married Jim that he would help me get satisfaction, that he would help me to feel good and respond. I just think it's his fault. I don't think he's really trying. I really think it's his fault.

Jim: Oh hell.

Laura: I don't think he really gives a damn. He says he does but I don't think he really does.

Jim: Why am I working the way I'm working?

Laura: Oh, you took me out of Chicago. You separated me from my mother and now you expect me to be, I don't know what to you. Like those girls you dated before, in bed all of the time.

Jim: It wouldn't have hurt you if you had done some dating before either.

Laura: Well, I did do some dating, and you put me down all of the time. What do you mean I didn't do any dating? You know damn well I did some dating. I didn't go to bed but I did date.

Dr. Lief: How many brothers and sisters did you have?

Laura: I had none.

Dr. Lief: You were an only child?

Laura: Yes.

Dr. Lief: Were there any unusual experiences, sexual experiences in your childhood?

Laura: No. We didn't even talk about sex, much less think about it in my house.

Dr. Lief: Jim, you're making a face, do you know something about this?

Jim: That is the coldest family that I have ever seen in my life. If they ever shake hands, that's great affection. Laura, you know that's true. She has never learned to love.

Laura: You're always talking against my family.

Jim: Well, look what they did to you.

Laura: What did they do to me? I think I'm pretty nice.

Jim: They made you a frigid woman.

Dr. Lief: Jim and Laura, we have to stop now. One of the possibilities is that there is a team of therapists out in St. Louis that have had a great deal of success treating problems of this sort and I would like you to seriously consider this as a possibility for treatment.

Jim: What's it going to cost, Doctor?

Dr. Lief: Oh, about $2,500.00.

Jim: My, God!

Laura: You earn enough. Don't you want to do it? Don't you want to try it?

Dr. Lief: Well, the two of you give this some more thought and certainly you are deeply concerned about this. That is abundantly evident so that since you are so concerned about your sexual and marital happiness this might be something that you might want to consider seriously.

Laura: Do you think that there is any possibility that I could be helped?

Dr. Lief: Oh, indeed. . . .

Laura: And that I could be normal?

Jim: Well, if they can help her, why it will be fine. It will be worth $2,500.00.

Dr. Lief: Well, I think before you can really get help, both of you have to see that it is an involvement with both husband and wife. Jim you are involved in this as much as Laura.

Laura: Thank you, Dr. Lief.

Jim: You mean I have to go through that, too?

Dr. Lief: Yes, you will have to. You'll have to see your part in this as much as Laura does.

Jim: I thought it was obvious it was her problem, Doctor.

Dr. Lief: You'll talk about that some other time.

The Couple Are Now Referred to Drs. Runciman and Doyle

Dr. Runciman: Let us tell you briefly where we are in this particular program. We will assume that at least three days have gone by. Our program is an intensive one, as you know. It has approximately 12 to 14 sessions. It's done on a daily basis, taking as much time as is necessary. With the particular couple on the first day, I will take the sexual history of Jim and Lee will take the sexual history of Laura. Following this Lee and I will come together, discuss the histories, listen to each other's tapes and decide what areas we still want to fill in. Then I will see Laura on the second day for more of her sexual history and Lee will see Jim.

Dr. Doyle: We take an intensive sexual history and are directive in asking specific questions. We do not say, have you ever masturbated? We do say, at what age did you start masturbating? At what age did you start sexual practice with the opposite sex? At what age did you have any homosexual activity? Assuming that this had been done.

Dr. Runciman: On the third day, we have a session in which we explain where they have been, why they think and feel as they do, explain where they are up to here and now, and what has to be done in order to achieve *their* goal.

Dr. Doyle: We give them an opportunity to defend or repute our statements in regard to our feelings about their relationship.

Dr. Runciman: At that stage, we explain that they have to work as a team on the problem. We would say to Jim, "This is not her problem, it is *their* problem."

Dr. Doyle: We have a two fingered approach—a team approach to resolving their difficulties in responding to each other.

Dr. Runciman: In order for us to help them we explain to Jim that he actually will be the one that will help Laura reverse her problem and each time, in the sessions, to follow that he suggests once again that he is "doing his job." We remind him that it is not a separate act between the two, but consistently a procedure in which they work as a team.

Dr. Doyle: It's *their* responsibility.

Dr. Runciman: At this stage we would have been through this and they would have decided that they have to go through the entire procedure of working as a team to reverse this problem. We know their sexual histories, obviously Lee and I will have to make a lot of assumptions. We have gone through their sexual histories, we've confronted them with how they are going to work as a team. Lee will tell you what we have programmed in terms of sensate focus or as Lee calls it—"pleasuring."

Dr. Doyle: As Dr. Runciman said, the first two days is history taking. The third day—round table. At the end of the round table as far as assignment is concerned, each of them is to touch each other from the top of their heads to the bottom of their toes, touching every area of the body that they possibly can—leaving no parts untouched except breast and genitalia.

We, the therapists, determine who initiates this beginning activity by the problem that is presented. With the nonorgasmic female generally we suggest that she initiate the stroking, the touching, the patting, the rubbing, the caring—in a physical way first. At that time I will ask Laura to start this with her husband at least two or three times in the next 24 hour period, the time length being as long as it is pleasurable to both. That's her responsibility. Jim's responsibility to Laura is to tell her what is pleasurable and what he likes most. Also he tells her what is not pleasurable in a positive way. "Laura this feels better than this," "Stroke a little harder," "Move in circular strokes," "Ooh that feels good." Some way, either verbal, nonverbal, body language, moving in and out, they both have responsibilities to each other. Laura to initiate, Laura to stroke, Jim's responsibilities feedback to her as to his feelings, desires, pleasures, etc.

Dr. Runciman: And no attempt at intercourse at this time.

Dr. Doyle: Also, avoiding as far as the female is concerned the breast and the genitalia areas. For the male, avoiding penis, scrotum, etc. That doesn't mean touch the stomach and then hop, jump to the leg. You can stroke through but not for actual sexual stimulation, just for feeling good.

Dr. Runciman: The other essential aspect of this is that they develop some kind of basic communication in which they tell each other what is pleasurable. There are many times, when they first come back to St. Louis, when they've tried intercourse on arrival in hope that they could resolve the problem on what would be the second honeymoon. We ask them not to have intercourse at all during this time and we also establish by this procedure the ability for them to literally talk to each other in bed, tell each other what is pleasurable.

Dr. Doyle: The communication concept of sharing—two days of pleasuring—one with no genital touching—one with genital caressing. Then, we will get feedback from those experiences. At the end of the fourth day then we program them into other positions, if it has been pleasurable, if it has been acceptable, if they understand it and being a pleasurable positive, not necessarily exceptional, sex isn't a negative, you know.

Dr. Runciman: We are now going to get the results. Today we

will see how the last sessions went as a result of using this "sensate focus."

Dr. Doyle: We would like to have a report, either one of you can begin, as to how you felt as you were being touched.

Laura: I liked it.

Dr. R.: What did you like about it, Laura?

Laura: Well, it felt good. It felt tender and it felt loving and I like that.

Dr. R.: Did you feel he was involved with you?

Laura: Umh! You will have to ask him about that. I wasn't sure. Part of the time I felt that he wasn't, I felt that he was just doing it.

Dr. R.: Just doing it because. . . .

Laura: Just doing it because you asked him to do it. He was being a good boy.

Dr. D.: How did you feel, Jim?

Jim: Oh, she puts me down but I felt very loving and I tried to be gentle.

Dr. D.: Will you tell her that?

Jim: You know, Laura, I tried to be gentle. I tried hard and you say it didn't work!

Dr. R.: Jim, you really felt that you were trying? You seem upset.

Jim: I tried very hard.

Dr. R.: You feel that you were trying to be involved?

Jim: And I was involved.

Laura: I wish I had known.

Dr. R.: You believe him right now, Laura, when he says this to you?

Laura: Yes, yes, I believe him now. But I didn't, I really didn't feel. . . .

Jim: That's the closest we have ever been. Not at all you didn't feel it?

Laura: I felt it a little bit but not very much.

Jim: Well anyway I tried.

Dr. D.: Laura, what could he have done to make you know that he really was in there trying?

Laura: I guess if he had really, if you had told me, if he had come across the way he just did now, I would have felt closer to you. You didn't.

Jim: No, I didn't, I didn't.

Dr. D.: This is so important to both of you to know that you are really enjoying it.

Jim: Well, I enjoyed it. It was the first time that she really has caressed me ever.

Dr. R.: How did you feel about her involvement with you, Jim, when she was caressing you, touching you?

Jim: Well, it was kind of hard for Laura.

Dr. R.: It was hard for Laura?

Jim: It was kind of hard for her. She isn't used to, you know, being free but I thought she tried to and I felt she was involved. Yes.

Laura: I was. I really was.

Jim: I felt so. It was really the closest you have ever been physically to me.

Dr. D.: Do you really hear what he is saying, Laura?

Laura: I hear. I feel very close to him now.

Dr. R.: That's a good feeling, isn't it?

Laura: Yes.

Jim: The best feeling we ever had.

Dr. R.: Good. Fine. Now you two are working as a team which, of course, is the whole basis we want—that of working together. We're pleased to see you two respond to each other that way. And of course you are finding out something that is basic to the whole purpose "to work as a team," to achieve your goals together.

Dr. D.: And Jim working back and forth.

Dr. R.: Jim, during this time that you and Laura were going through this procedure, did you have erections?

Jim: Yes. And, we talked about whether we should try to have sex but we thought maybe it would be better to wait. I wanted it very much but we thought we should. . . .

Dr. R.: "Follow the instructions," since we asked you not to.

Jim: Yes.

Dr. R.: Laura, how about you? Did you notice any increase in lubrication, or feelings at all?

Laura: Some, some. Not all that much. Some, but it's really hard. It's still hard. I guess I'm still scared.

Dr. D.: How did you feel when you approached him? Did you notice a difference?

Laura: I was scared. I was really scared. I didn't know how he was going to respond and I didn't know whether I was doing the right thing and I felt clumsy about it.

Dr. R.: Well, did you understand, Laura? You said you weren't sure whether you were doing the right thing. Was he telling you the things that were pleasant to him?

Laura: Some of the time. Some of the time he was. Maybe he needs to tell me more.

Dr. D.: That's very reassuring to be told, isn't it?

Laura: Yes.

Dr. R.: How about you, Jim? Did you feel that you know what Laura liked when she was being touched?

Jim: I asked her. Yes.

Dr. R.: You asked her?

Jim: Yes. It is kind of hard for us to talk about things. We never really talked before except to blame each other, I guess.

Dr. R. to Dr. D.: Shall we take them to the next part of the program?

Dr. D.: Yes.

Dr. R. to Dr. D.: All right, why don't you take them into the next step.

Dr. D.: All right, since this has been pleasurable and since there are some, you know, moments of awkwardness and so forth, but obviously each of you are trying, we would like to suggest something else. Since Laura is lubricating better, and having some more warm feelings toward you, Jim, we would like to put you in a different position and we would like for you to actually stimulate the clitoris. We've requested that you not touch the genital areas and breast areas. Still we do not want intercourse. Jim the position for you is to put your back at the headboard, legs separated. Got it?

Jim: Yes.

Dr. D.: Laura, scoot right up to him, buttocks up to stomach, legs across his legs, actually separating your legs, with your head back against his shoulder in a comfortable position. There all ready?

Laura: Yes, I'm there.

Dr. D.: This gives Jim a complete accessibility to the body, incorporating the sensate focus, touching all over, but from around behind you, stroking inside of your legs because you said earlier that was pleasurable. Then he also has easy access to the clitoris. One thing we want to warn you about, Jim, is to be sure that lubrication of the vaginal tract is used because you know Laura has complained that you hurt her and if you lubricate the clitoris well, with vaginal lubrication or saliva, it won't hurt.

Dr. R.: And Laura, you must tell Jim at all times. In other words, you can actually take his hands, you see, and help him in placement, and speed and movement, and the amount of pressure because Jim has no way of knowing unless you actually tell him, verbally or with body language. You can either do that by using your hands or telling him in any way so that he knows what to do to bring you pleasure.

Laura: I'll try, I'll try.

Dr. D.: Actually, Laura, you can be very much in control of Jim's movements which give you pleasure. If you get uptight, uncomfortable, or he gets grabby as you say, you can just stop him so that you can relax.

Laura: That's all right if I stop you?

Jim: Yes. Let me ask something. I thought women liked aggressive men and now you are kind of putting the girl in charge.

Dr. D.: Your time will come. She is not telling you "what to do" but "what things bring pleasure to her."

Dr. R. to audience: In co-therapy, whenever the question is raised by the male, it's the female co-therapist who answers the question in terms of a woman. If Laura asks me a question, I answer her in response from the male standpoint and those of you already doing co-therapy would agree that once you work this way, you don't want to work any other way when you are working with couples with sexual difficulties so notice how the questioning will go.

Dr. D.: I want to add to my statement of your time will come.

Why I mention this is that Jim, we stated earlier that giving and receiving is very important. And right now we want each of you to learn to receive and you to give. Sometimes in our culture, giving and receiving are very difficult to learn because the man is taught to be the giver in sexual activity and the woman is taught to receive.

Jim: Huh, huh, all right.

Laura: Will you not hurt me?

Jim: Well, I've never wanted to hurt you. I never have. Maybe you can tell me if I hurt.

Dr. R.: There's no way Laura that he can hurt you because as long as you two are communicating, you have a constant way of telling him exactly what is pleasurable to you so there is no way that he can hurt you now. You two have worked at it, establishing the communication process in which you can respond to each other in terms of letting each other know.

Laura: I guess I needed that.

Dr. R.: And you understand, Laura, you respond in any way that you choose in terms of telling Jim, by gesture or by movement. That of course is very pleasurable to Jim because he knows that he is giving you pleasure and that is the essential thing that you two are working at now as a team in giving each other pleasure. Giving has its own reward.

Dr. D.: Do you want to give to her, Jim?

Jim: I've always given to her.

Dr. D.: Do you want to continue?

Jim: Yes, that's why I'm here.

Dr. D.: Will you tell her?

Jim: Laura, I want it to work and I'll try to give.

Laura: Thank you.

Dr. R.: And, Laura, you want to do the same thing for Jim, don't you?

Laura: I want to try and I want to give to you, too.

Jim: Laura said that she had a little lubrication. I wonder if we are ready for that yet. Whether we shouldn't have maybe a couple more nights when we just stroke rather than what you are suggesting, whether that's too frightening to you.

Laura: I—I—I think I am scared.

Dr. R.: Well, certainly there is going to be a certain amount of fear of this because you seem to be concerned that maybe we are moving too fast, but at the same time you must remember you have a control of each other. You can mutually agree at any moment if it is too much pressure for you both. We want you to move at your own pace, at your own speed, working together. So don't have a fear that you may be pushed into something because you can now tell each other when you wish to more or less slow down and go back.

Dr. D.: The only thing we are asking is no intercourse tonight and the other depends upon you.

Jim: There is no fear about that, I think.

Dr. R.: Well, we'll take them into the next session.

Laura: Before we go, you know, I didn't like that. I don't know what you meant by that. And that makes me feel bad.

Jim: What makes you feel bad?

Laura: I felt as though you were putting me down. Were you putting me down?

Jim: What did I say?

Laura: You said that there is no fear about that, about intercourse.

Jim: No, because I just said I didn't want to move too fast, Laura. I said that the time before. I just meant I didn't want you to go too fast and we wouldn't try what we shouldn't. I wasn't putting you down.

Laura: But the way you said it.

Dr. R.: You two don't have to worry about the speed of the program because we have gone through this many times with many couples and we will set the pace for you.

Dr. D.: I guess they should go ahead and communicate about that because Laura doesn't understand and he is trying very hard to tell her what he means.

Jim: Well, what I simply was trying to say was that I don't want to go any farther than you can go. I didn't mean to say it hostile, mean, okay?

Laura: Thank you. Okay.

Dr. D.: Laura, do you understand?

Laura: Yes.

Dr. R.: Let's assume that they have had that session. Let's get the report, okay? Following day, all right?

Dr. D.: Good morning.

Laura: Good morning.

Jim: Good morning.

Dr. D.: How do you feel?

Jim: Well, I guess we made some progress, but it didn't go very good.

Dr. D.: How's that?

Jim: I'm not being mean, honey. Laura just has problems in responding. She turns off.

Dr. D.: Tell us about it.

Jim: Well, we of course caressed, and then I tried to caress the clitoris and she got kind of tight like that and told me that what you said was you weren't ready for that, and I tried to be understanding about it.

Dr. R.: How were you understanding? What did you say or do?

Jim: Well, I said to her "all right honey." And then we tried again later on in the day.

Dr. D.: Besides what you said, what did you do?

Jim: I quit but of course I was disappointed because. . . .

Dr. D.: Okay, stop right there. Laura, checking out on that, when he said "Okay, Honey," would it have helped anyway if he had patted you on the bottom or stroked your legs. . . .

Laura: Anything, anything. If he had just reached out and held me like that.

Dr. D.: Okay, would you tell him how and what you would have liked from him when you got uptight.

Laura: When I was like that, Jim, what I really wanted you to do was just to take me in your arms and say it's all right, it's all right, you don't have to respond, it's all right.

Jim: Well, I wanted to do that, Laura, but I felt as I have felt for two years, I felt so rejected and we are here and we are trying and another rejection. Even though I knew I should, I couldn't. I just felt rejected and bad.

Laura: You felt rejected.

Jim: Yes, because you turned me off.

Laura: You felt rejected the night when I couldn't respond to you?

Jim: Yes, you were turning me off, Laura. I know you were trying.

Laura: But it was me, it was my fault. I wasn't. . . .

Dr. D.: Wait, please, today is the first day of the rest of your lives. As long as you refer back to negative experiences, you will find it difficult to move forward.

Jim: But that's pretty hard to leave every—we've had two years of frustrations.

Dr. R.: Remember our goal when all four of us mutually agreed that we would have to change the pattern. You were in a pattern and you revert back to it from time to time. The point is you don't have to keep reverting back. You have a new base which, you listen to each other and overcome particular situations. Jim, do you understand what Laura told you? How she could have felt comfortable if you had just responded in that way, does that make sense to you from her standpoint?

Jim: Yes, the words make sense but what I am saying is I had feelings.

Dr. R.: But what about your feelings, Jim? Were you able to get them out at that time?

Jim: No, I guess not. I guess I didn't tell you about them.

Laura: No, you didn't.

Dr. R.: Did you just not feel like trying to tell her, you felt it hopeless, or . . . ?

Jim: I felt a little angry and discouraged and. . . .

Dr. R.: And you weren't able to tell her those things?

Jim: No, I guess not, I guess I didn't.

Laura: You made me feel very bad. I was feeling bad to start with when I couldn't respond and then you made me feel worse.

Dr. R.: I think you both know what you should do. We have given you a way to overcome it. You can do it yourselves by telling each other your feelings. You said later on in the afternoon you tried again. What happened that time?

Jim: Was it better?

Laura: I wouldn't say so.

Jim: Or did you just do it?

Laura: I just—by that time I just felt awful. I just felt there was no use and that we might just as well not try.

Dr. D.: Jim, did you know this?

Jim: No, I didn't understand that. I would have quit if I had understood that.

Laura: Well I felt as though I should do it. That that was part of the plan and I hadn't done it before and I hadn't responded right before and should try.

Jim: I thought you liked that.

Laura: Oh, I didn't really.

Jim: You didn't?

Dr. R.: Laura, remember we told you at the beginning of the program that as long as you two are continuing to work as a team, really nothing can go wrong. You see you preset yourself for failure by your concern that it didn't work this morning and it's not going to work again this afternoon. Now remember, you can always turn back to the touching and the feeling. You don't have to go through a procedure that is uncomfortable for you or you have a fear of at that time.

Dr. D.: There are really no errors. You will feel and touch when you feel good and feel bad. There are no mistakes.

Laura: That makes me feel better.

Dr. R.: It is only the general direction of the relationship. It is not the fact that you have to have success at one particular time. Even in your future sexual life together, there will be times when it will not be particularly gratifying for you, and at other times for Jim, but as long as you are working together as a team you have the right direction.

Dr. D.: Laura, you know you arise each morning feeling different. Interested in going somewhere. Ohooo I hate to think of those dirty dishes. The same thing applies to sexual response. Sometimes it's great, other times, oh let's don't. It is important to learn to say "no" and to say "yes."

Laura: I guess I was feeling as though I had failed. Somehow, I just wasn't measuring up and I couldn't do it.

Dr. R.: Laura, you are never failing as long as you are trying to work together, then you are in the right direction. There are no mistakes. If any problems arise in terms of some of the things we ask you to do, that's a learning process. You are learning it together. It's not a matter of failure at any time, Laura.

Dr. D.: Sex and sexuality is a big ballgame and we want you to take down the goal posts. First downs, water breaks, time outs, running up and down the field and even penetrations can be fun, not only the touchdown or score.

Dr. R.: Another day—another time. In other words we will assume that it is a day later and, Laura, in this case you have begun to have some new feelings. You are not orgasmic yet, but you are beginning to have very "new feelings." Now follow the procedure as Dr. D. and I use the building process of capitalizing on the positive aspects of the relationship so that we can keep moving them along. Now Laura, let's assume that you have had a good day and you come back into the office the following—in other words a good evening for response. And Jim you are proud because you know you have really been able to help her in this and things are moving along quite nicely. Now you may notice that Dr. D. and I may not share quite the high enthusiasm. We'll see how it comes out. All right Laura, how did it go last night?

Laura: Oh gee, it was great. It was just marvelous.

Jim: It really was?

Laura: It really was. I found myself having all kinds of feelings that I never had before.

Dr. R.: New feelings for you, Laura?

Laura: Yes, Yes they were. They were just great.

Dr. D.: Did you tell Jim this?

Laura: Oh yes.

Dr. R.: How were you able to tell him. How is the communication going now?

Laura: Oh I told him.

Jim: Oh tremendously.

Dr. R.: How did you feel, Jim, when she told you about these new feelings?

Jim: I felt very wonderful, but she really didn't have to tell me because there was the kind of moving towards me. A kind of feeling that we both felt. And then something else happened. When we went to dinner, I think for the first time, we really began to talk about all the other things about our marriage. Now, I think, Laura, for the first time I began to realize what I had done to you with all those long hours and leaving you alone. I really haven't been so thoughtful as I thought I was. We got it all out on the table and it was wonderful.

Dr. R.: In other words, you were finally having the success together working as a team that you were able to talk about some of the other aspects of your marriage.

Jim: Yes. Yes.

Laura: And he understood.

Jim: And you did, too.

Dr. D.: And then you understood, right?

Dr. R.: Jim, you say that you knew Laura was experiencing new feelings. How did you feel about this? Did it make it possible for you to be more inventive, to try more things? How did it work for you?

Jim: Well, I told Laura this, that really the marriage has meant to me—it's been kind of a defeat and I blamed her but I really felt inadequate. So what I really felt when she responded was something good about myself. I can't quite put it in words but I felt better, kind of like a man.

Laura: Yes, I. . . .

Dr. R.: Actually, you know what you two are telling us? That you are sharing your feelings and as a result of your sharing your feelings and building together that there are no limits. Is that what you get from this, Dr. D.?

Dr. D.: Pretty much so.

Laura: Well, I was feeling that, Jim, that you weren't using me, that you weren't taking advantage of me and that I meant something to you. That you really cared.

Jim: I felt the same way. I really did.

Dr. D.: That puts such a different aspect on the picture, doesn't it?

Dr. R.: Laura, what did you want to bring to Jim at that particular moment? Not only the fact that you were, of course, bringing your new feelings to him, but what were some of your feelings, maybe in addition to that?

Laura: Well, how much I really cared for him. How much he really means to me and how much I value you and how great I think you are.

Dr. R.: Is that what you talked about at dinner?

Jim: She told me.

Dr. D.: Did you find it easier touching him?

Laura: Hummm.

Jim: We've been touching all of the time.

Dr. D.: Then, you found it easier, though, that now you are more aware of Jim's value to you, you are not as apprehensive about touching him with this warm feeling of intimacy.

Laura: Oh no. I can't keep my hands off of him.

Jim: Laura is something else. I had a lot of girls but I haven't told Laura any of this, but I really wasn't very close to any of them and last night was the first time I really got close. It was wonderful!

Dr. D.: One thing before we end this session. We are going to end this session, aren't we, Dr. R.? This has been a beautiful day. Yesterday you were a little different weren't you Laura?

Laura: Yes.

Dr. D.: Remember, it may be a slow building process. You may hit a low but you can always think about tomorrow and the opportunities that you bring to each other.

Jim: It seems to me now that that isn't quite as important as it was. You know—the sexual part of it. We want to work it out but I think that the feeling that we caught is really rewarding in itself and the other way, it will work.

Dr. R.: Are you saying to us that even if Laura is not orgasmic you still feel you have got something going now that. . . .

Jim: We didn't have before. That's what I'm saying.

Dr. R.: You realize, Jim, that by telling Laura that she doesn't have to be orgasmic for you to have a good relationship, you have now given her the best opportunity to become orgasmic by taking the pressure off her for orgasm and as a result now you allow her in every sense of the word to have all of the feelings that you want to bring to her and that she wants to bring to you and experience for herself.

Jim: That's what I am saying.

Laura: I can be normal.

Jim: Yeah.

Laura: Thank you.

NOTE: This only includes the first few steps of the sexual therapy program.

Chairman: Now we have questions from the audience.

Question: I would like to ask a question about your last moments with the couple in which you more or less promised them that the wife soon would become orgasmic. I wondered if you—well that's the way I would have interpreted it and I wondered if you wanted to leave yourself open to that.

Alex: Well as you may notice we never promise anything, we only suggest to them that the potential is always there but note the emphasis on the woman to take the pressure away from her for orgasm. And, of course, they did such a good job in role playing that by Jim's wording, we have a whole new relationship anyway. That's essential to the program that the pressure is off because many of the wives are pushing for it, we have to work overtime in therapy to stop pushing for it. Orgasm has to happen spontaneously.

Question: In your first interview you focused on the mutual sensate communication. As you moved along, in later interviews, the way I got it was the husband was concentrating on fondling his wife and she was not doing the same beyond the first day.

Lee: In our program sensate focus is always used before any other traditional activities are programmed. A loving warm relationship which can be created by touching pleasurably including breast and the genitalia. That's the starting of both partners and is essential to sexual satisfaction in later activities. Loving, holding, touching, and stroking are all means of developing communication of feelings.

Alex: They also have a base line all of the time to see if things in the program have been moving along. They can always return back to the sensate focus because that is workable to them already. That has been established with them.

Lee: And remember, we do not emphasize the word "turn back" even though we are saying it here. Sometimes they feel as though they are regressing. We just note that this is one step and this they have done successfully so rely on it. And do it again, and then we'll go on to something else.

Question: In Sensate Focus, is this all strictly verbal or do you demonstrate and have this participate in some structuring and training in this physical involvement?

Alex: No, we don't have to, because we tell them two things (1) to be inventive as possible and (2) to be as imaginative as possible. But we might spend an hour and a half on that so they bring their own imagination to us as a result of exchanging with each other as to what is pleasurable. There is no demonstration on this.

Lee: One oddity, of course, about the subject of sexuality is that you have a list of erogenous zones which has been published and those lists do not hold true for each person or individual. One couple that Alex and I had worked with the man found that when stroked between his toes he was very stimulated sexually.

Question: Laura presented herself as a woman with primary frigidity, she has never had orgasm. Under what circumstances would you work with a woman alone with self-stimulation, masturbation, or with a vibrator, or any other technique that she can achieve orgasm by herself? Is that ever done?

Alex: Let me clarify your question. You mean they have come to us as a couple?

Question: They have come as a couple but instead of working together as a team you might have the woman stimulate herself. Is that ever done?

Lee: Yes, it is done by discussion—not by our observation, even with Jim present. We, of course, in the sexual history find out how much she has stimulated herself and what she has found out for herself to be pleasurable—what parts of her body and types of touching brings her excitement.

Alex: Right, the other thing is that we explain to Laura that she is the only human being who can find out actually what is pleasurable to her. Now in order to bring this to Jim she has to find herself by herself and then in turn transfer this information to Jim so that he in turn can bring this to her. In other words, it is a constant pursuit of what is stimulating. And once they are involved in the program they get very excited about finding out about themselves.

Question: I understand that the premise of your therapy is the general relationship of patients and doctor, in other words, they are coming in with a helplessness that they are both facing. You are exhorting, clearly setting out for them a defined program which will surely lead to satisfaction. How often do you encounter a kind of your patients, which I felt growing in me sitting here to what came across as an absolute sureness that your method and the therapist, I'll be damned if I am that sure 90 percent of the time, and it bothered me that there could be a relationship between four human adults in which there was a clear cut line that would always be making you the authorities, they would always be the help of infants, and they would always be rewarded by you for the success of the day after. They come back. . . .

Lee: You're feeling it too much. I'll try to answer this in saying that such a response to both of you is a learning response, it is a natural process but a learning response. We are trying for them to relearn about their sexuality without sexual intercourse being their only goal.

Alex: Also, I want to say that both Lee and I share your feelings. I can only assure you that we found it workable and we were only after results. We certainly share your feelings about our apparent assurance. But that actually is a part of the program that we found successful. Just remember, that we never deal in this particular program on how to raise children, how to set up a family budget, we bear directly on the sexual problem and that is the approach that we use. You are correct, we are the authority figures. We are directive as you say. I had the same feeling when I first trained because of my own background and training.

Lee: Two weeks is the time limitation we have with the sexual program.

Question: Say the patients are already in psychiatric therapy and the patients thereby have someone with whom they have an ongoing relationship outside, do you do the same sort of thing with them?

Alex: Yes. We will take them, as many of them come to us who are in ongoing therapy. It is better to have a neurotic male who is potent than a neurotic male that is impotent. It is better to have a neurotic female that is orgasmic than to have a neurotic female who is not. (We only take couples when the other clinician endorses our therapy.)

Alex: I would like to give our couple an opportunity to describe some of their own personal thoughts about this particular interviewing session.

Laura: One of the things that concerned me a little bit was when you described, Lee, the position that I was to take in bed with Jim, at that moment in my role and my mind I got this image and the image was a frightening one at that time. Now, I being a timid and kind of, you know, inhibited and restricted kind of person, would not share that with you so that I kept that image in my mind and I think that partly that would have militated against a spontaneous reaction that night. Now, would you give me an opportunity had I been your patient, had we really been patients at that time, to kind of explore this? Would you have elicited other kinds of things?

Lee: I would have asked "How do you feel at this particular moment. Do you feel comfortable? What are your feelings now that I'm asking you to do these kind of activities?"

Alex: And remember, Laura, she would have programmed you into it but I as the male therapist (when you began to express some concern) would immediately remind you how important it was, and I would use the term "If I were Jim" sort of thing and how much you are giving me by opening up and, we have already gone through your conditioning process and told you that many things are now acceptable. We have pretty well conditioned you to have a whole new approach which you are excited about. So you actually are trying and the more you do and the more involved you become, the easier it becomes for you.

Lee: Okay, accepting the fact this is an awkward position. . . .

Jim: I don't think it's awkward.

Lee: Don't speak for Laura.

Jim: Let me make one comment about my reaction to the therapists. I agree in terms of our emergence into all kinds of new experiential relationships in therapy. But, in one session they were saying to me "now don't try to have intercourse tonight." And I said "Well, there's no chance of that." I was being extraordinarily hostile and Laura picked it up. They, I felt, smoothed it over. We weren't given an opportunity really to deal at this time with our feelings and I got away with a rationalization of that which was dishonest. What I am really saying to them is that if the structure is so rigid that it doesn't give opportunities to pay attention to the kind of emotional feedback, it's going to interfere with the structure then it's just too damned structured. See. On the other hand, on one occasion, they had a conference between themselves when Lee said "I think Jim and Laura ought to work that out." I felt relieved that you felt with me enough at that time so that my emotional discomfort could have been brought out. What I am saying is that there is a rigidity sometimes to structure. You do this this day and this this day and because it has been before rewarding, you then forget that the great agenda is the patient and I felt sometimes your agenda was a schedule and not the patient.

Lee: We aren't really that way, Jim. We were so interested in getting across our techniques and our time was running away with us. . . .

Jim: All right.

Alex: And Jim, I want to say to you, I couldn't agree with you more. I remember the moment but as Lee says it was our concern of limited time. We normally would stop right there and would have had that brought out right there with as much time as necessary because we are not structured in the fifty minutes and that would have been resolved right there.

Question: The question I have bears directly on this. We saw in the first interview that Laura had a fear of pregnancy and childbirth. Is it possible and let's suppose that it was also true that she had a fear that sex was a violent act and that she would be harmed by it. Would you have taken up the fears in your therapy or would that have been left completely aside?

Lee: We would have taken it up. I think, Alex, at the round table, wouldn't you?

Alex: Most assuredly. At the round table it would be a good question. It would be continuous, not only at the beginning but right on through reminding her all the time of these original feelings as to how it affects her. Remember, Lee you want to see her alone, or I would want to see her alone. We would break it any time you would want to. Because it's not as structured as it may appear. We would take the individual situations and work with them as they develop.

Lee: And we have this opportunity for reminding her because it is only typical that you bring up your past, your past experiences. No one can start today to go forward without considering his past experiences.

Jim: May I ask one question? In the beginning I came in, as you must have been aware, extraordinarily frightened and anxious and therefore expressed it hostilely. And I am not sure at the end of that hour that I didn't feel kind of turned off in dealing with that because Dr. Lief turned to my wife and talked with her about her problem. I didn't feel that hostility really was dealt with so that I could want to come back because I was made to feel more comfortable and I wonder. . . .

Alex: I was aware of that. In other words, we weren't dealing with your fear, anxiety, your feelings of rejection. It was just limited time. If there had been more time we would have taken this up.

Chapter XII

COUNSELING TECHNIQUES: CASE STUDY DESCRIPTION

Joseph N. Mertz

W HEN I WAS APPROACHED to make a contribution to Therapeutic Needs of the Family, my first reaction was affirmative, since I have always felt that there was a real need for a practical, down-to-earth approach to the problems which many counselors encounter in Marriage Counseling. After I gave an affirmative response in terms of contributing material to this book, I became rather apprehensive when confronted with the task of attempting to present counseling sessions which would give the reader some insight and working knowledge about an actual case. The case which I have selected is not unique. However, it is a case that has many facets of disturbances and one that illustrates quite clearly how previous marital failures and disturbances can and do influence future marital ventures and the adjustments which both husband and wife are called upon to make if some measure of happiness and success is to be achieved.

CASE STUDY OF ALBERT AND CAROL E.

This is the case of a young couple known to me since April, 1971 and seen in regular weekly therapy sessions for a period of one year, after which therapy was gradually decreased until currently they are seen every three months on a maintenance level. Albert is 32, a graduate engineer and formerly married, divorced from first wife in 1969 and is the father of three children from that union, all girls ages 9, 10, and 12. Carol is 27, an RN by profession, formerly married for a period of four years, divorced 1969, no children by her former marriage. This couple were married in December, 1970, after a courtship of a year and a half. Premarital sexual relations were entered into with some guilt response on behalf of Mrs. E.

221

Mr. and Mrs. E. were referred to my office by their minister. The problems were multiple and surfaced almost immediately after marriage. These were centered in what Mr. E. described as his wife's emotional state, "She's always upset. I'm afraid to say anything to her." He felt that she was scared of him and told her that she was foolish to feel like this. Mrs. E. on the other hand felt that she could not live up to her husband's expectations, she felt that he was continually making comparisons between his first wife and her. She admitted being fearful of speaking her mind to him and as a result communications broke down at all levels. An additional major complaint on behalf of Mrs. E. was her husband's lack of attention at an affectional and sexual level. These feelings were further highlighted by Mrs. E's desire to become pregnant and later learning that she was sterile. Adoption plans are now being worked through.

This abbreviated account of the presenting problems gives an indication of the multiplicity of problems confronting this couple. The therapy or counseling sessions cover a span of a year and a half. Initially sessions were on an individual basis, with joint sessions every four or five weeks. As insights were developed and the relationships stabilized, joint conferences were substituted for individual sessions.

The First Interview

When I first met this couple, I was impressed by their apparent genuine concern for one another and their marriage as a whole. I saw Mrs. E. first and then her husband; these individual sessions being followed by a joint conference. This process which for reasons of clarity I shall designate as a Diagnostic Session, normally takes an hour and a half. Usually I have only the barest of essentials regarding a case and so must rely entirely on this initial contact to give me as concise and well-rounded a picture as possible of the presenting problems.

Both Mr. and Mrs. E. were somewhat apprehensive as to what they had to expect in this initial meeting, since neither had ever sought professional help in the past. However, with the basic introductions out of the way and with direct and warm support on the therapist's behalf, they were able to relax sufficiently to describe in detail their attendant problems.

In order to give the reader a proper format for the interviews that follow, I shall briefly outline the certain things which I hope to accomplish in such an initial contact with a patient or patients.

A. I first identify myself and attempt to answer any questions directed to me, and make known that since I am a therapist and the patient is experiencing difficulties (as in this case), that there is a professional reason for our meeting together.

B. I attempt to obtain basic facts by direct questions, providing the patient is not too apprehensive or agitated. This includes how the patient views his problems.

C. I make it clear to the patient that there are no restrictions on use or choice of words or expressions of feelings, providing such expressions of feelings are not harmful to patient or therapist.

D. I usually do not attempt to offer interpretations in the initial session unless feelings and reactions are of such distortion and of such proportion that an interpretation might assist the patient to view the problem in a more realistic way.

E. I conclude the initial interview by outlining my plan for therapy, presenting the patient with a generalized schedule of meetings, setting fees for services, and discussing finances if this is indicated. The need for mutual cooperation is stressed in terms of maintaining a regular continuity of therapy sessions if positive results are to be achieved. I hold out no carrots or no magic wand. I feel that this is extremely important for the patient to understand and accept.

The Second Interview: With Mrs. E.

Th: Hello, Mrs. E. How do you feel today?

Pt: Mr. M., do you think that you can help my husband and me? I know that I love him, but I'm not quite sure how he feels about me.

Th: What do you think makes you say that?

Pt: (Pause) I'm not sure. How can I ever be sure if Al never wants to talk to me? It seems that I'm the one who has the problems. He's so arbitrary, he's the boss, he makes all of the decisions. At times I feel completely wrong and yet I know that I'm right—at least I think I am. (Long Pause) I guess I'm frightened. (Long Pause)

Th: Frightened?

Pt: Yes, frightened. I keep thinking that Al and I will go our separate ways and then once again I'm a failure.

Th: (Pause) Do you see yourself as a failure because of your first marriage?

Pt: Yes.

Th: Would you like to tell me about it? (Pause.)

Pt: (She then describes her first husband, how he drank, his cruelties and emotional outbursts and his refusal to have children. This return to her past was accompanied by a varied display of emotional reactions; crying and fidgeting in her chair.)

Th: Do you really feel that you can compare Al with your former husband?

Pt: (Pause) No, not really. I guess not. That's what attracted me to Al. You see he was my patient and he was always so kind and considerate not only of me but toward the other nurses and orderlies who came into his room. Well, he was so different and I never was used to being treated like I was a person with feelings. (She then went into detail of their courtship and how kind and gentle Al was with her. She talked of their sexual involvement and how she was the aggressor rather than Al and how afterwards she felt guilty—not because of the sex—but she felt that perhaps she trapped Al into marrying her.)

Th: Perhaps you feel like this because of your present inability to communicate your feelings to Al.

Pt: Perhaps so, but he always seems so withdrawn, I really feel trapped. I just break down and cry. I know that he resents me when I do this, but I can't help it. (It was here that Mrs. E. first indicated that she was the one who initiated the idea of counseling and her husband's rejection toward such help.)

Th: Do you feel that your husband doesn't see any real problems in the marriage?

Pt: I really can't say for sure. I believe that he realizes that we have problems, but I also feel that he perhaps thinks it's all me.

Th: Are you saying that he doesn't see his contributions or involvements in his relations with you as a factor?

Pt: I guess so.

Th: Can you as a person see where possibly you are creating some of the present disturbances?

Pt: (Pause) Well, I'm not sure. Perhaps, I'm afraid that I can't live up to what he expects of a wife.

Th: What does he expect?

Pt: I don't really know. I do know that he's bitter toward women on account of his former wife. She deserted him and took his three children with her. He don't like to talk about it, but from what I know, he came home from work one day and found the house deserted. You had better ask him. He might be more open with you.

Th: I intend to discuss this with your husband. One thing you both must learn to realize is that I can only help you as far as each of you want me to. It means that we must learn to trust one another and each of you must feel free to discuss feelings openly. What may seem unimportant to you might be one of the keys we're searching for. Building bridges to closer communication will enable each of you to become more sensitive to each other's feelings and needs in a more realistic and objective way. It will help each of you to gain a deeper understanding of one another. Once this happens, changes in your relationships will gradually emerge.

Pt: I feel that you're right. Anyway, I do feel better just knowing that we're doing something.

(End of Session)

The Third Interview: With Mr. E.

(Mr. E. came to my office accompanied by his wife who waited in the waiting room. Both were chatting amiably together.)

Pt: I noticed your sign on the door says psychotherapist. Could you tell me what psychotherapy is and will you do it with us? How does it work?

Th: I'll be happy to explain this to you. It's not as complicated as it may seem. (I then proceeded to explain in some detail what psychotherapy was and how it could be related to their problems being as these problems were generating some inner emotional response.)

Pt: You say that such therapy will help us to untangle our feelings and relate better to one another. Am I right?

Th: Yes, in some respects you are right. However, movement up or down will depend on how you and your wife are able to respond to the guidance and direction which you will receive from our sessions. If you are able to remain free and open in your approaches to the problems within the marriage, gradual insights will be developed, enabling each of you to become more aware of each other's personal needs. You must attempt to realize that many problems within marriage emerge solely because either one or both of the marital partners either tend to attempt to live isolated from one another or go to the other extreme of attempting to change their spouse into what they as a person feel a husband or wife should be. Neither of these approaches to marriage can work successfully. Marriage should not deprive a person of his individuality, rather it should enable a man and woman to join forces for the greater good and wholeness of both as a unit, but still keeping the individual nature of each intact. I hope that counseling and psychotherapy will do just this for you and your wife. I also realize that you will become angry at times and be in disagreement with what I say. I want you to feel free to express your feelings in the way most comfortable to you. Do you feel that you understand?

Pt: Yes, but I must admit that I have a lot of questions in my mind, but when I'm here I can't seem to recall things.

Th: This is understandable. But, why not try and jot down things that you perhaps want to talk about between each visit.

In this way some of your questions as well as your anxieties can be dealt with, so that you will feel more comfortable.

Pt: That seems like a good idea now, but later on I feel really foolish. Tell me, just how would you describe me?

Th: It's interesting that you should ask me this, since I'm quite interested in how you see yourself, not only as a person but in your relationship with your wife.

Pt: Not very much I'm afraid. You see, I'm still trying to figure out why my first wife left me. We never had any serious disagreements; well, at least not what I would call serious. I really thought that we had a good marriage until I came home and found her gone without any word of explanation. I can't tell you how I felt or for that matter how I feel. In fact, I'm still in the dark.

Th: Perhaps I can help you to clear up some of the feelings which you have regarding your former wife. It would appear that with some of the feelings being generated within your present marriage, that the same or similar factors contributed to the breakdown of your former marriage. In other words, whether you realize it or not, your behavior and attitudes were a contributing factor in the decision made by your first wife to leave you.

(A Long Pause)

Pt: (Somewhat Angry) I don't need you to tell me that I drove her away. God knows that I tried to be a good husband and father. If she was so miserable, why didn't she tell me? (Pause.)

Th: Perhaps she tried to communicate her feelings to you in ways other than by talking. I really don't know, but perhaps as we progress in therapy reasons for past events might become more clear to you.

Pt: Maybe you're right. (Pause) Well, I know you're right in what you say; if you weren't, I wouldn't be having problems in this marriage.

Th: I think it's good for you begin to come out of yourself, but try and remember that marriage is a continual interaction of two people and the breakdowns within marriage are the results of both people malfunctioning and not just one. So, try not to be too hard on yourself.

Pt: Just one thing more before I go. (Pause) Will you tell me what to do to make this marriage come out OK?

Th: Well, not in so many words. A lot will depend on the situations between you and your wife and how things develop during the course of therapy. Certainly, I'll provide guidance to each of you and when the occasion warrants it, I'll present alternative courses of action. However, my main role will be to help both you and your wife to gain insight into yourselves as individuals, thereby, enabling each of you to view each other more objectively so that each of you can reach a level of maturity where your individual choices and decisions will achieve some measure of happiness and compatibility rather than dissension and grief.

(There was a brief discussion and the session was terminated.)

Reflecting on these first three interviews, the reader can fairly well visualize the interactions between patient and therapist and the various psychotherapeutic approaches which were utilized. Fortunately, in this case illustration, we have a young married couple who are well-educated as well as being highly intelligent. They came to therapy with some awareness that problems existed and from the onset recognized the need for professional assistance. With these factors present, it was fairly safe to predict a favorable prognosis for this marriage on an overall level.

In succeeding interviews with both patients, they were able to develop personal insights into their own individual self and gradually become aware of how they were reacting to each other under specific conditions which faced them in day to day living. Mrs. E. originally presented fearfulness of her husband's reactions and had previously attempted to relate to him as she felt that he would want. Such an approach put her on the defensive and when positive responses from her husband were not forthcoming, she experienced feelings of rejection and at times much hostility which she attempted to cover. By the same token, Mr. E. rejected his wife's advances for fear of letting down his defenses and possibly placing himself in a vulnerable position; something he was determined not to do.

The therapist assumed an active role and helped each person to view his/her individual self as he/she existed in the eyes of the other. The gradual self-awareness that emerged enabled each to feel more secure within his and her self as a person in their normal interactions with one another. Physical, emotional, and verbal responses increased, facilitating communication at all levels. With these new feelings of inner security permeating their relationship, both Mr. and Mrs. E. were gradually able to enter into and resolve problems which heretofore they tended to repress or at best handle on a superficial level.

As therapy progressed new problems were uncovered and it's interesting to see how these were dealt with. The three children of Mr. E's first marriage became a real threat to Mrs. E. for she realized that sooner or later she would find herself in a person to person encounter. The normal concerns of a stepparent were further enhanced by her own feelings of being in competition with Mr. E's first wife. In effect, she felt that no matter what she did in her relations with the children, some degree of criticism would be forthcoming. The first such encounter was during the children's summer vacation when they came to visit their father and stepmother for a period of two weeks.

The following interview brings out some of Mrs. E's feelings with reference to this initial visit in August.

The Nineteenth Interview

Mrs. E. came to the office looking fresh and cool in spite of the hot humid weather which we were experiencing. She seemed relaxed and greeted me in a friendly way.

Pt: I have a lot to talk about. Al's children are with us and while it's not as bad as I first thought it would be, I'll be glad when the next week is over and they return home. I seem to be getting along with them famously and we seem to have fun together, until their father walks in. Then, I'm totally ignored and they do exactly what they feel like doing whether I approve or not. (She then went on to describe an incident where she laid out the children's clothes for church. The end result was that they refused to wear what she selected. Rather, they went to their father and had him select the clothes. Mrs. E. reacted to this by telling them to wear what she put out for them, expecting to have her husband's backing. The outcome was that Mr. E. sided with the children, saying his wife was making a big fuss about nothing. While describing this incident Mrs. E. became quite emotional and alternated between a display of anger and crying. Then she stated quite simply, "I'm telling you all of this because you had advised me of possibly having incidents similar to this and because you seem to understand. I certainly wish Al had some of the same understanding for my feelings.")

Th: I'm sure this must have been difficult for you. But since you yourself recognize that we had previously talked of such possible reactions on behalf of the children as well as of your husband, why do you permit your feelings to get so out of control?

Pt: I don't know. Somehow I've been trying so hard to make it a pleasant time for the kids as well as for both Al and myself, then I seem to wind up with a kick in the rear end.

Th: You're human.

Pt: At times I don't feel like it.

Th: How do you feel?

(Long Pause)

Pt: Tired of competing for Al's affection and tired of trying to break through to him.

Th: But, a few weeks ago, you agreed that there have been a lot of breakthroughs and changes. In fact, you even recognized that you are changing in many ways.

Pt: I know, but it all seems to futile at times. I guess I'm a bit upset. All I want is for Al to see me as a person, my feelings, my needs as his wife. I also want to give him children, but I guess that will never happen. He loves children and I'd feel better if we had a child, but I just can't seem to get pregnant.

Th: Do you see children as a bargaining point for Al's affection? Is this why you want a baby?

(Pause)

Pt: No, not for that. I guess I felt cheated in my first marriage. I really don't feel that a woman is complete unless she's had a baby.

Th: I think I understand.

(Patient began to cry. Pause of about five minutes.)

Th: Perhaps in our next meeting we can talk about this, since it seems quite important to you. There are ways to work this through and I'll help you.

Pt: I'd like to talk more about it, but I know we can't now, since my time is almost up.

Th: Well, I feel that we should attempt to work one thing through at a time. You will still have the children for another week and perhaps things might start going better now that the ice between you is broken. I think that you should try and realize that strangeness and some apprehension also exists on the children's behalf and on your husband's behalf as well as your own. One such meeting will break the ice, but it will take more get-togethers in the future for all of you to feel comfortable and really build up close personal interactions and relations.

I'd advise you to freely talk over your feelings with Al and perhaps you might even agree to accompany him to his conference with me, so that the three of us could have the opportunity to talk over the feelings which you both are experiencing at the present time.

Pt: I'll try and follow through on what you advise, and I'd really like to talk out my feelings with you and Al, if Al doesn't mind my coming with him. I'll certainly speak to him about it. You know, I always feel better after our conferences, and I know that I can work this out. Both Al and you will be proud of me.

(End of Session)

As therapy continued, both Al and his wife brought out how their relationships were growing and developing with Al's children. In fact, Carol met Al's former wife on several occasions and while no deep relationships were established, the former Mrs. E. began to accept Carol's sincere interest in the children and no longer attempted to put barriers in the way of the developing relationships between the children and Carol.

Gradually, this couple have developed insight into each other's needs and currently they are successfully working out existing problems. Therapy has been reduced to every three months at a maintenance level. As previously stated, adoption plans are being completed, since it has been medically determined that Carol is unable to have children.

In this case presentation, all modes of counseling were utilized from time to time. As a therapist, I have always adopted a strong role whether it be supportive or active counseling. It's my firm belief that we cannot permit patients or clients to flounder in the morass of their own inadequacies and the confusion resulting thereof. The therapist has a prime responsibility to guide, direct, and channel the thinking and energies of the patient into avenues which will lead to the goals and aspirations which he has set for himself.

In connection with this, I would like to present some basic criteria which in my opinion a therapist, counselor, or any practitioner working with patient or client problems should possess. I cannot accept the premise of some of my fellow practitioners who attempt to do therapy by the book. A therapist should be a vital dynamic being throughout the entire therapeutic process. He should be able to participate with the patient as well as playing the role of observer, depending on the overall therapeutic field and the interaction which may or may not be generated. He should be able to adequately deal with shifting areas of focus, even though there might be little advance evidence of the shifts about to take place. Certainly, a therapist should also be skilled in the art of nonverbal communication in terms of the individual nature which his client or patient presents during the course of therapy. No therapist should ever attempt to mold a patient in his or her concept of what a patient should be, do, or react to. The individual should be encouraged to develop within his own framework of reference and in a manner comfortable to himself.

From time to time, the therapist should evaluate his own responses and reactions to the patient. He should be able to feel comfortable within a therapeutic situation wherein both dependency and independence are alternately experienced so that independence can be gradually fostered and with proper guidelines therapy can be gradually reduced and eventually terminated as the patient accepts more and more responsibility for his own actions as a person.

Collaboration with other professionals should be a prime commandment of every therapist. It's very easy in practicing on one's own, to fall into complacency and to permit individual personal needs to color our approach to the patient's problems. In reexamining our own motivations and gaining objective approaches from our colleagues, both the therapist and the patient will benefit.

INDEX